ACUPUNCTURE RISK MANAGEMENT

The Essential Practice Standards & Regulatory Compliance Reference

David C. Kailin, L.Ac., M.P.H.

CMS Press   Corvallis, OR
1997

Acupuncture Risk Management
The Essential Practice Standards
& Regulatory Compliance Reference
By
David C. Kailin

© 1997 David C. Kailin

All rights reserved. No part of this book may be reproduced or transmitted in any form or by any means, electronic or mechanical, including photocopying, recording or by any information storage and retrieval system without written permission from the author, except for the inclusion of brief quotations in a review.

First Printing: 1997
Printed in the United States of America
Publisher: CMS Press, a subsidiary of
                 Convergent Medical Systems, Inc.
                 P.O. Box 2115
                 Corvallis, OR 97339 USA

Cover Design: Old Town Graphic Design, Corvallis OR
Printing & Binding: McNaughton & Gunn, Inc., Saline MI
Printed on Acid Free paper for longevity.

Library of Congress Catalog Card Number: 97-80443

Kailin, David C.   1948-
Acupuncture Risk Management
The Essential Practice Standards
& Regulatory Compliance Reference
CMS Press, Corvallis, OR, USA
Includes bibliographic references and index.
ISBN 1-891426-00-1
1. Acupuncture.   I. Title.

        97 98 99 00   10 9 8 7 6 5 4 3 2 1

Table Of Contents

Introduction		5
1.	Dimensions Of Risk & Benefit	9
2.	Scope Of Risk Management	19
3.	Contexts Of Risk	27
4.	Physical Plant	31
5.	Employers & Employees	47
6.	Bloodborne Pathogens	57
7.	Records & Billing	77
8.	Medical Advice	99
9.	Medical Emergencies	111
10.	Interpersonal Aspects of Treatment	117
11.	Legal Aspects of Treatment	125
12.	FDA Regulations	141
13.	Technical Aspects of Treatment	151
14.	Acupuncture Needles	159

15.	Moxibustion	177
16.	Cupping	187
17.	Coining	197
18.	Herbs & Dietary Supplements	207
19.	Acupressure	219
20.	Electroacupuncture	227
21.	Laser Devices	235
22.	Magnetic Devices	245

Appendices			251
	A.	Form & Record Examples	253
	B.	OSHA Hazard Communication 29 CFR 1910.1200	281
	C.	OSHA Bloodborne Pathogens Standard 29 CFR 1910.1030	297

Resources	311
Bibliography	315
Index	329

INTRODUCTION

This book is primarily intended to train acupuncturists to assess many dimensions of risk, and to implement practical strategies for the prevention of harm. More generally, it guides all complementary medicine providers toward practicing safely in the social, legal and medical contexts of America. You have selected this *wake up call* to help you examine - and possibly transform - every aspect of your practice. While your livelihood certainly depends upon it, so might your life.

Standard acupuncture texts, often translations or adaptations of Oriental reference works, present the student with the conceptual and technical bases for Traditional Oriental Medicine (TOM). These texts contain the essence of the traditional technical art, including certain aspects of safety (e.g. maximum needle insertion depths). But defining safe techniques requires broader frames of reference than TOM.

With the transition of acupuncture to America, several key elements of praxis have been left understated (if not entirely unstated). Among these are issues of how to proceed in the contexts of American medicine and culture. Failure to grasp prevailing healthcare, legal and personal expectations can directly lead to adverse outcomes. Risk management extends well beyond technical safety.

Acupuncturists are accountable to prevailing local standards of medical practice and judgment. Yet were acupuncturists to hold nothing but local standards, they would have naught to offer. The clinical value of acupuncture derives from it's foreign perspectives and inherently 'other' practices. Acupuncturists must achieve a delicate balance, distinguishing greater from lesser medico-legal risks in the meshing of Oriental and American practice standards. The task involves subtle levels of judgment, acquired with added difficulty by those individuals lacking prior biomedical professional experience in this culture. Effective risk management requires educated discernment.

Until recently there seemed little need to attend to such issues, as acupuncture occupied a liminal place in America, marginalized enough to be well ignored. Acupuncture's profile has risen, with the mainstreaming of alternative therapies into medical institutions and reimbursement plans. Regulatory bodies have discovered the need to make accommodations to assimilate acupuncture. Acupuncturists find themselves increasingly answerable to surrounding medical and regulatory communities. The transition from alternative to orthodox is a challenge for all involved.

The essence of that challenge is to carry the living art of acupuncture within the contexts of American medicine. In response, acupuncturists need a strong background in biomedical standards of practice, and in the legal and regulatory framework. On the bright side, those practicing at standards broadly accepted in American medicine will realize enhanced employment and reimbursement opportunities. Acupuncturists not planning on basic regulatory compliance might as well start planning for a different career. Readers will find the status of this transformation of standards of practice reflected throughout the text.

At the outset, the text indicates that helping, harming, safety and liability are deeply intertwined subjects spanning technical, legal, medical, ethical and social domains. Basic concepts of risk management are then presented. Those perspectives inform a detailed examination of risk and strategies for risk reduction in ten functional contexts of a generic acupuncture practice. Summaries of 'Best Practice' recommendations conclude those chapters dealing with technical aspects of risk.

Located in the Appendices are pertinent form and record examples, and two key Occupational Safety & Health Administration (OSHA) regulations. To help you keep abreast of changes in the federal regulatory environment, a list of agency Internet web sites is provided in the Resources section. (Computer literacy is yet another facet of our increasing engagement with American culture!) Readers accessing the Internet and literature citations will find the text is a touchstone to a continuous process of self-education.

I am fortunate to have learned very little of the subject matter by personal experience of untoward events. Yet this project has spurred me to radically revise my own clinical protocols. Medline searches provided adverse effects evidence to ponder. Representatives of professional liability insurance companies thoughtfully outlined aspects of claims experience. OSHA and FDA personnel contributed invaluable advice and detailed explanations. Thanks are extended to those who attend my seminars and graciously share difficult clinical experiences.

Profound gratitude for the insights of Karen Chase, Caroline Heaviland, Alex Holland, Anna Manayan, Neal Miller, Barbara Mitchell, Margaret Naeser, Mark Nolting, Michael Pope, Martin Shaw and Dennis Tucker, among other fine guides. Thanks as well for the mentoring and forbearance of friends and family. With talented input many errors have been avoided; those remaining are solely the author's responsibility.

Given the vagaries of individual legal circumstances, the author and publisher recommend consulting a lawyer for specific legal issues. This text presents federal regulatory requirements to the best of our understanding, but official policy may differ. OSHA regulations in particular vary by state. The text does not broach state regulatory requirements. Consult state and federal regulatory agencies for official policy and compliance guidance. We cannot guarantee that the information herein will be sufficient for your compliance requirements.

Suggested clinical protocols need to be assessed and adapted to your setting, and deemed fit in your professional judgment. For specific advice on biomedical issues, consult a medical doctor. The text presents educational information and is intended neither as individual legal counsel nor medical advice. The mention of a company or product does not constitute endorsement or advertisement. The author and publisher will not be liable for direct or indirect harms resulting from any uses of the material contained herein. If these conditions are unacceptable, promptly return this text to the publisher for a refund of the purchase price.

What has been learned in hindsight is offered to enrich your foresight. You will be challenged time and again in these pages to assess your work practices, and to train (or re-train) yourself to proceed in the contexts of American culture. Meeting this challenge is essential, if we are to manifest the abundant benefits of acupuncture in mainstream American medicine, now and throughout the 21st century.

David C. Kailin
October, 1997

Chapter 1

Dimensions Of Risk & Benefit

A discussion of ethics frames entry to an appreciation of multiple dimensions of risk and benefit. From the principles of 'Do No Harm' and 'Do Good' we develop a statement of accountability to minimize risks and maximize benefits fairly across a moral community. The 'cascade of risk' demonstrates widening consequences of adverse events.

Ethical Contexts

Every health care provider shares two moral principles: 'Do No Harm' and 'Do Good'. These are remarkably different goals, and at times they conflict. Providers attempt to do good by applying their training in diagnostics and therapeutics to decrease pain and suffering, and yet this simultaneously increases the potential for several types of harm. Among harms are the side effects of treatment, delay in seeking other forms of care, the psychologic burdens that may accompany diagnostic labeling, and (reading the term 'harm' most broadly as any cost) the patient's time and financial expense for services. In practice, preventing harm and providing help are not mirror images of each other. The 'goods' often reside in different dimensions than the 'harms'.

Preventing harm and providing help merge seamlessly in the clinic, and yet involve separate strategies of enactment. Devising an initial treatment, acupuncturists may select fewer points to needle, and stimulate the needles less, to gently introduce patients to the sensations. This provides a graduated experiential education for patients, to decrease the harm of perceived fear. Yet the points selected are therapeutic for the presenting medical problems, drawn from a strategy of helping. In this example, a strategy of helping is modified by a strategy of preventing harm. Acupuncturists engage in these calculations almost unconsciously.

The idea is to generate balance between the competing goals of preventing harm and providing help. Should preventing harm become overly dominant, the resultant practice might be known (in a pejorative sense) as 'defensive medicine'. In this instance, the patient bears excessive costs of preventive strategies, when the primary beneficiary of risk reduction might well be the provider. On the other hand, should providing help greatly dominate, one would heedlessly incur a variety of excess risks and increase the likelihood of iatrogenic harm - those adverse events caused by healthcare provider intervention.

The concept of moral community is relevant to several succeeding points. A moral community consists of those entities to whom one owes a duty. **Table 1.1** offers a general outline of an acupuncturist's moral community, with elements listed roughly in order of nearest to most distant. What does your moral community look like? What are the risks and benefits to each member?

Acupuncturists contend daily with decisions relating to the allocation of goods and harms across a moral community. When planning the nature and extent of treatment for a patient, we attempt to balance the interests of: the patient and their family, the acupuncture profession, contiguous professions, legal and regulatory agencies, insurers, and our own costs and benefits. As a result of allocation decisions, goods and harms are unequally distributed among entities in the moral community.

ELEMENTS OF MORAL COMMUNITY

* Self — Family, Community, Sacred World

* Patients — Families, Communities

* Employees — Families, Communities

* Employers — Families, Stockholders

* Co-Workers — Contiguous Professions

* Profession — Local, Regional, National, Global

* Insurers

* Regulators

Table 1.1

Additionally, notice the asymmetrical reciprocity of duties in the moral community. The obligations we have toward one party are different in quality, quantity and time occurrence than the obligations that party owes us. Consider the duties a patient has toward a provider - to arrive at appointments timely, to pay for treatment, to report on symptoms, to accept some discomfort of treatment. Quite different than the duties of a provider toward a patient (which will be dealt with at length later).

In clinical practice, performance of duties is not an entirely static matter. While some obligations are held invariably, others are prone to situational revision. There is a tendency to honor duties to more distant elements of a moral community with greater selectivity. Yet those distant elements may expect full compliance at all times. For example, the U. S. Food & Drug Administration (FDA) expects all herbal preparations and medical devices on our premises to comply with their standards. Now had acupuncturists complied with the FDA's longstanding definition of acupuncture needles as experimental devices, they would not have engaged in the clinical practice of acupuncture until the 1996 revision of needle status! Irrespective of any antipathy engendered by that earlier ruling, acupuncturists must conscientiously weigh their responses to each FDA-imposed duty. We are part of the FDA's moral community and they are part of ours, and so in various ways we are mutually accountable.

Accountability refers to something more than responsibility. Accountability is a non-transferable obligation. One might delegate to an assistant the responsibility to remove needles, but in the event of a needle accidentally left *in situ*, one cannot delegate away personal legal accountability. Accountability is role intrinsic. Society defines duties for health care providers, and providers internalize those duties as they learn a professional role. In contrast, responsibility is more extrinsic in nature. (Porter-O'Grady 1996)

Now examine this fully developed statement of our task in relation to the principles of Do No Harm and Do Good: <u>We are accountable to minimize risks and maximize benefits, and to allocate these equitably, across our moral community</u>. Each acupuncturist develops implied, working risk/benefit and fairness calculations, based on their individual understanding. Those calculations must incorporate prevailing standards of practice from both within and beyond the acupuncture profession. Prevailing standards of practice are often implicit. In the course of this text, many standards will be stated explicitly.

Dimensions Of Risk

An understanding of the dimensions of risk is a necessary precedent to effective interventions involving them. A number of dimensions become apparent upon considering the expanding sequence of harms in the *cascade of risk*, presented in ***Table 1.2.***

<u>Material harm</u> is in a primary sense equivalent to physical damage to a body. An accidental pneumothorax is an unequivocal material harm. Material harm may be extended as a dimension of risk to include the legal concept of battery, broadly meaning any unauthorized touch. It may also be extended to include psychologic harm, offense to the sensibilities of the person before us. Finally, consider excessive monetary costs to the patient as a secondary form of material harm. Material harm is often the entry point to the cascade of risk. It includes dimensions of additional pain, suffering and costs to the patient and their family.

CASCADE OF RISK

* Material Harm
* Perceived Harm
* Relational Failures
* Consumer Legal Actions
* Regulatory Actions
* Personal Repercussions
* Societal Repercussions
* Professional Repercussions
* Transferred Risk Repercussions

Table 1.2

Perceived harm involves much more of the interpretive dimension, in placing significance and meaning on material harm. Perceived harm is demarcated from material harm by its greater variability through individual construction. What is dismissed as insignificant harm in one context - subcutaneous extravasation of blood down the forearm secondary to a blood draw at a hospital clinic - may be perceived as significant in another context - the coining bruise at an acupuncture clinic - although both share a similar visual appearance, similar degree of material harm, and similar causal basis in arising from an intent to help. Indeed, there have been cases of coining bruises on children mistaken as signs of child abuse, with referrals to child protective service departments.

It is not just that harm may be perceived as significant by interpretation, for there are also biases in the attribution of fault, and in the consequences, or liabilities, for perceived harm. The cultural legitimacy of mainstream medical practices is such that many avoidable adverse outcomes are accepted without attribution of fault. Despite licensure in most states, acupuncturists in America do not have the protection of a deeper cultural legitimacy to buffer attribution of fault and ensuing liabilities.

Relational failures are the hinge upon which material harm and perceived harm swing, activating deeper levels of the cascade of risk. In the presence of a warm and authentic relationship between patient and provider, much is shared, understood and forgiven. Lacking that, little may be forgiven. Malpractice attorneys advise building good relationships with patients to generate significant protection from professional liability torts. Relational integrity also contains remarkable therapeutic potential for patients and providers.

Consumer legal actions commonly arise from the triad of material harm, perceived harm and relational failures. Practitioners may be sued for damages resulting from accidents involving their premises as well from breach of their professional duties. Such actions are costly in terms of money, reputation and prolonged angst.

<u>Regulatory actions</u> may be initiated by complaints made to licensing and other regulatory agencies. Agencies also initiate actions in the absence of complaints, based on evidence of a practitioner's lack of statutory or regulatory compliance. In addition to monetary penalties, one's license to practice may be at risk of limitation or revocation. Ignorance of regulatory requirements is a substantial risk factor.

Repercussions from the above events are wide ranging. At the <u>personal level</u> one can expect major expenses, loss of income and reputational damage. Defendants commonly experience feelings of shame, guilt and loss of self esteem in relation to their moral community.

At the <u>societal level</u>, when stories circulate concerning adverse experiences with acupuncture, people are led to miscalculate acupuncture's relative risks. Material harm caused by acupuncture is still exotic enough to be newsworthy.

At the <u>professional level</u>, tragic errors - particularly foreseeable and avoidable errors - have the potential to negatively impact every practice in a wide area. We are mutually reliant on each other's impeccable performance.

Ramifications at the <u>level of transferred risk</u> refers to effects on professional liability insurance companies. Excessive claims cause malpractice insurance rates to increase, and can eventually lead companies to withdraw from the market. Without malpractice insurance, access to hospitals and other medical facilities is denied to the profession.

The dimensions of risk include, but clearly transcend, material harm from technical error. Physical, psychological, perceptual, relational, legal and regulatory risks each entail different strategies of prevention. Acupuncturists are called upon to proactively control the entire range of risks. That involves the functions collectively known as risk management.

CHAPTER 2

SCOPE OF RISK MANAGEMENT

We define risk avoidance, risk control and risk selection, and then briefly present the functions of risk management. The chapter closes with a look at the incidence and nature of patient material harms.

Risk Management

In large corporations, the functions of risk management are divided among specialized professionals. Acupuncturists usually manage all aspects of risk in concert with their other duties. Effective risk management requires a working knowledge of risk management functions. Several basic terms are first defined.

Risk avoidance is the creation of conditions for the total absence of a risk. The exclusive use of pre-sterilized disposable needles, used once and then immediately discarded into a sharps container, entirely prevents the potentials for patient-to-patient disease transmission associated with re-usable needles. This is an example of risk avoidance which simultaneously induces few other risks.

Risk control means decreasing the frequency and/or severity of harm. Risk control strategies are applied in instances where risk avoidance is not possible or practical. Gloving the hand that holds the cotton ball just prior to needle removal decreases - but does not entirely prevent - the practitioner's blood contact infection risk. Risk of infection via accidental needlestick, among other events, remains possible.

RISK MANAGEMENT FUNCTIONS

* Risk Assessment

* Risk Control Planning

* Risk Control Implementation

* Risk Control Communication

* Risk Monitoring

* Risk Financing

* Crisis Response

Table 2.1

Risk selection involves the linked choices of 'which risks to incur' and 'which risks not to incur'. One must choose preferable sets of risks. For example, installing a smoke detector decreases the risk of damage to property and life from undetected fires. Yet it simultaneously increases risk of damage from false alarms. Imagine smoke from indirect moxibustion setting off the alarm, and the possibility of several patients with needles in place responding in panic. As is frequently the case, the control of one risk induces other risks. When risks cannot be avoided altogether, select for preferable sets of risks. In the above example, the practitioner could substitute infrared lamps for moxa poles, controlling the risk of false alarms by reducing smoke production. But this induces risks of the lamp tipping over, and of being placed too near the skin. With each risk control selection, the set of resultant risk reductions and risk inductions must be evaluated anew.

We turn now to a brief examination of risk management functions (Head 1989), summarized in **Table 2.1.**

Risk Assessment concerns identifying the nature and location of risks, establishing (when possible) their causes, frequency, severity and costs.

Risk Control Planning involves analyzing and selecting risk avoidance and risk control strategies for assessed risks, and developing an implementation plan to reduce risks.

Risk Control Implementation means putting a risk control plan into action. This may involve some or all of the following interventions:

 * safety-related administrative policies
 * re-engineering of the work environment
 * re-design of tools
 * re-design of work practices

* use of personal protective equipment (PPE)
* provision of immunizations
* use of safety devices
* employee risk control education programs
* risk monitoring
* risk financing

<u>Risk Control Communication</u> concerns the initial and periodic training of employees in risk control rationales, policies and procedures. It includes communicating with employees about actual and potential adverse events that occur in their workplace.

<u>Risk Monitoring</u> involves recording the occurrence of adverse events and high-risk situations, particularly after implementation of a risk control plan. Employee compliance with risk control efforts may be monitored. Risk monitoring provides informational feedback for a continuing process of risk control planning.

<u>Risk Financing</u> typically involves the transfer of certain risks through insurance. Acupuncturists often need two types of insurance: premises liability and professional liability. Premises liability insures equipment and furnishings in case of damage from fire, burglary, etc. It also covers claims arising from injuries occurring on the premises, such as might result from slipping on a loose rug. It does not cover injuries directly caused by acupuncture treatment. Professional liability (malpractice) insurance covers claims arising directly from acupuncture treatment. Policies often contain exclusions for specified techniques or conditions. Read the policy carefully to understand what is covered, and what is not.

<u>Crisis Response</u> involves preparations for effective response to specific types of emergencies. Common emergency preparations might include fire, burglary, earthquake, electric power loss,

computer failure, computer security breaches, and medical emergencies.

The scope of risk management is indeed broad. Yet each acupuncturist, of necessity and in ways both formal and informal, fulfills the many duties of a risk manager.

Incidence & Nature Of Patient Material Harms

For many dimensions of clinical risk, important outcomes are practically unquantifiable. For example, one senses but cannot easily measure the ebb and flow of relational bonding with patients. The incidence and nature of material harms to patients are particularly difficult to establish. Malpractice insurance claims constitute the primary data applying to the question of incidence of harm - 'how often do material harms occur'. Claims and medical journal articles also contribute to the question of 'what sorts of material harms occur'.

An insurance executive shared the following figures: from a risk pool of approximately 1,200 acupuncturist policyholders, an average of two claims per month arise, resulting from about four reported adverse incidents per month. (Anon 1996) Assume each claim is brought against a different acupuncturist (i.e. that multiple claims are not clustered around just a few individuals). Also assume that the policyholders represent a cross section of the skill levels of the profession, much like a random sample. Finally, assume there are 10,000 practicing acupuncturists in the USA. (This figure is from a 1996 informal tally of licensed acupuncturists, and presumably includes relatively few M.D. and D.O. acupuncturists). One could then estimate that this segment of the acupuncture profession faces 200 claims per year, based on 400 adverse events. The data suggests that about 4% of acupuncturists per year experience a significant adverse event in their practices. A Norwegian study estimated an adverse event occurs every 4-5 years in each acupuncture practice there. (Norheim & Fonnebo 1995)

However, the assumptions are terribly flawed. Perhaps the most risk averse practitioners carry malpractice insurance, while the most incautious forgo it. In that event, the data would underestimate adverse incidents. But even more telling is this fact: for all types of medical practices, unreported adverse incidents vastly outnumber reported incidents. Accurate estimates of the incidence and severity of harms cannot be made from available data.

What sorts of material harms have happened to patients? An uncritical review of malpractice insurance claims, medical journal reports, and summaries of legal and regulatory actions has been used to construct **Table 2.2.** Selections of related medical journal articles are cited in Chapters 14 and 18. Readers are encouraged to consult and periodically monitor the medical literature for acupuncture adverse events. (See Internet Medline in Resources.)

Given the limited scope of what comes to the attention of insurance companies and medical journals, one cannot conclude that Table 2.2 presents the only patient material harms occurring to date.

Of course, patients are not the only potential recipients of material harm. Acupuncturists are at risk of contracting Hepatitis B (HBV), Hepatitis C (HCV), the AIDS virus (HIV), and other bloodborne infections in the course of work. (See Ch.6, Bloodborne Pathogens)

REPORTED MATERIAL HARMS

Bacterial Endocarditis
Billing, Fraudulent
Bruising
Burns, Accidental (Cupping, Ind. Moxa)
Cardiac Tamponade
Delayed Biomedical Care
Epidural Hematoma
External Ear Infection (Press Needle)
Fainting
Gastroenteritis
Hepatitis B Infections
HIV Infection
Needles, Broken Accidentally
Needles, Imbedded Intentionally
Peripheral Nerve Damage
Pneumothorax
Sexual Misconduct
Spinal Cord Lesions
Subarachnoid Hemorrhage

Table 2.2

The record well supports the contention that <u>significant material harms related to acupuncture can happen, do happen...and could happen in your practice</u>. Hence prevention is an essential duty.

Statistical data are inadequate to the majority of risk assessment needs. Acupuncturists must develop an innate sensitivity to potential risks, guided by medical, legal and social experiences from the medical professions.

Having briefly narrowed the focus to patient material harm, we now return to a multi-dimensional understanding of harm. The concepts and functions of risk management will be applied to ten distinct contexts of risk in acupuncture practices.

CHAPTER 3

CONTEXTS OF RISK

Ten contexts of risk are introduced: Physical Plant; Employers & Employees; Bloodborne Pathogens; Records & Billing; Medical Advice; Medical Emergencies; Interpersonal Aspects of Treatment; Legal Aspects of Treatment; FDA Regulations; and Technical Aspects of Treatment.

Contexts Of Risk

Contexts of risk refers to risks arising from the diverse functional aspects of an acupuncture practice. The contexts of a somewhat generic practice employing one or two acupuncturists will be presented. There are, however, a great variety of practice settings (solo, group practice, HMO, hospital, etc.) and employment arrangements (self employed, professional corporation, employee, contractor). Adapt the examples to develop risk assessments and risk controls suited to your workplace. Herewith are ten salient contexts and the ground of their attendant risks.

In the context of Physical Plant, Chapter 4, are risks arising from aspects of the clinic premises and its contents. This includes building security; ADA (Americans with Disabilities Act) access requirements; HVAC and electrical systems; fumes, vapors and particulates; fall injuries; OSHA (Occupational Safety and Health Administration) emergency action and fire prevention plan regulations; and OSHA chemical hazard communication rules.

In the context of <u>Employers & Employees</u>, Chapter 5, we introduce employer's basic duties; hiring & firing; policies & procedures; the provision of optimal ergonomic work conditions; and the implications of accepting the conditions of work.

In the context of the OSHA <u>Bloodborne Pathogens Standard</u>, Chapter 6, we present requirements for employers to develop and implement an Exposure Control Plan. The employer must define methods of compliance involving specific engineering and work practice risk controls, informed by the concept of Universal Precautions. An HBV vaccination program and a post-exposure evaluation and follow-up plan are mandated. Hazard labeling, employee training, and recordkeeping are also addressed.

Arising from the context of <u>Records & Billing</u>, Chapter 7, are risks associated with medical record contents; record confidentiality & release; and record retention & destruction. Treatment limits & billing limits; ethical billing practices; and collection practices are next presented. The chapter closes with a review of procedure codes; and diagnostic codes as related to scope of practice.

The context of <u>Medical Advice</u>, Chapter 8, broaches issues of the advice given at the initiation of provider/patient relationships; scope of advice as related to scope of practice; guarantees of outcome; the informed consent process; diagnostic & prognostic labeling; and professional relationships.

In the context of <u>Medical Emergencies</u>, Chapter 9, we define common medical emergencies and discusses the need for response protocols and first aid supplies. The chapter closes with discussion of the limits and imperatives of first aid response.

The context of <u>Interpersonal Aspects of Treatment</u>, Chapter 10, brings issues of the therapeutic relationship; rapport; privacy & modesty; and sexual boundaries.

In the context of <u>Legal Aspects of Treatment</u>, Chapter 11, we address scope of practice; the nature of explicit duties; negligence; primary care provider status; and the dilemma of non-standard medicine & standards of care.

In the context of <u>FDA Regulations</u>, Chapter 12, we review FDA medical device regulations, and then apply them to acupuncture devices. The chapter closes with an evaluation of dietary supplement regulations.

The final context, <u>Technical Aspects of Treatment</u>, is examined in detail over ten chapters. Chapter 13 serves as the prelude, in which we comment on the nature of the technical guidelines; define 'Best Practices'; explain equipment sterilization & disinfection protocols; and mention other basic hygienic & safety practices.

Succeeding chapters discuss risks and risk controls related to Acupuncture Needles; Moxibustion; Cupping; Coining; Herbs & Dietary Supplements; Acupressure; Electroacupuncture; Laser Devices; and Magnetic Devices. These chapters conclude with 'Best Practices' as brief recaps of risk control strategies.

In our standard format, we will first define *Risks*, then present a *Discussion*, and close with a concise review of *Risk Control Strategies*. Proceed to the first context of risk, Physical Plant.

CHAPTER 4

PHYSICAL PLANT

In the context of Physical Plant are risks arising from aspects of the clinic premises and its contents. We consider building security; ADA (Americans with Disabilities Act) access requirements; HVAC and electrical systems; fumes, vapors and particulates; fall injuries; OSHA emergency action and fire prevention plan regulations; and OSHA chemical hazard communication rules.

You might be seeking a location for your new acupuncture practice, or perhaps you have already established an office. Your concern with risk management begins here, assessing the physical plant, its surroundings and its contents. Some of those concerns are shared by OSHA, while yet others are addressed by ADA regulations.

Building Security

Risks:
Crime related physical harm and property damage.

Discussion:
Clinics exist in and are subject to a social context that includes criminal activity. Assess crime risks when determining the location of your clinic. Then consider interventions to help control the risks. If your personal mission is to serve in a high-crime area, such risk controls are all the more crucial.

Risk Control Strategies:
Locate office in low crime risk area. Ask other tenants, neighboring businesses and police about local crime experiences.

Ascertain that parking areas, entryways and hallways are well lit.

Install a secured entrance (e.g. intercom & electronic lock release), and/or a security alarm system.

Obtain premises liability insurance policy.

ADA Access Requirements

Risks:
Lack of handicapped access; ADA regulatory compliance.

Discussion:
Handicapped access is more than a nicety - it is a requirement of Title III. of the Americans with Disabilities Act of 1990. Under that code, medical offices are regulated as 'public accommodations'. Removal of barriers to handicapped access in existing facilities is required, when readily achievable to do so. If it is not readily achievable, then the practitioner must identify an alternate way of serving handicapped patients, if it is possible to do so. New construction and all remodeling must incorporate handicapped accessibility. Parking areas, curb and step ramps, entryways, hallways, bathrooms, drinking fountains and public telephone placements must all be designed to accommodate wheelchair users. Civil penalties for a first violation of the ADA may not exceed $50,000.00. Both the landlord and the tenant are considered to be liable for compliance, but the responsibility may be allocated between them in the lease. (DOJ 1992; CBBBF 1995)

An office on a very steep sidewalk, despite other access features, might effectively impede or endanger handicapped access (particularly in inclement weather). Consider this factor in selecting your clinic location.

In addition to physical access, providers must accommodate diverse communication needs for persons with vision, speech, hearing or cognitive impairments, if that is possible without undue burden. If a relay telephone service for the deaf is not available in your locale, consider installing a TTY (text telephone). (NRH 1994)

Risk Control Strategies:
Assess building location for safe handicapped accessability.

Assess wheelchair access from parking areas to the office.

Assess wheelchair access to a restroom with a transfer bar equipped toilet stall, and with a sink for seated users.

Determine and make readily achievable changes.

Negotiate a clause in your lease allocating responsibility for any premises-related ADA compliance costs that may arise.

If a relay telephone service for the deaf is not available, consider installing a TTY (text telephone).

HVAC & Electrical Systems

Risks:
Malfunctioning heating, ventilation, and air conditioning (HVAC) systems and electrical systems.

Discussion:

HVAC systems maintain suitable working conditions, and in failure can bring the clinic to a halt. Heating systems can present fire and carbon monoxide hazards as well. Preventive maintenance and alarm systems are of the essence.

Concerning electrical systems, care should be taken to avoid overloading electrical circuits. Long runs of extension cord can overheat. Inspect electric cords to determine that they are not frayed or worn. Test electric outlets for functioning ground wires (you may need an electrician to do this). Building codes require grounded outlets, but older buildings may not have been brought up to code.

Risk Control Strategies:

Confirm or arrange for regular maintenance of heating and cooling systems.

Clearly delegate responsibility for maintenance and repair in the lease.

Install smoke detectors and carbon monoxide detectors.

Inspect electrical system and correct detected problems.

Don't overload outlets.

Use only fused power strips if additional outlets are needed.

Obtain premises liability insurance policy.

Fumes, Vapors & Particulates

Risks:
Illnesses from fume or vapor inhalation, or excessive particulate matter in the air.

Discussion:
Odors emanating from new carpeting, carpet backing, mastics and glues, paints and finishes, exhaust fumes and solvents may contribute to 'sick building syndrome'. Molds and low air exchange rates are also factors. Exposure reportedly makes some people acutely ill, and others chronically ill. It is prudent to recognize the risk of such exposures and avoid locations with detectable chemical or mold odors. Modifications in ventilation, accelerated off gassing, and/or replacement of synthetic carpets may remedy the problem. (Uppsala Univ. Hosp. 1997; OSHA 1995)

Fumes from moxa can cause headaches in some, and the smoke and odor can be a nuisance to staff, patients and other building occupants. Consider alternatives to indirect moxa, such as infrared lamps. (See Chapter 15.)

OSHA regulations apply to particulates in the air, as chronic inhalation of dust-sized particulates can irritate the lungs. When working with herbal materials, there may also be questions about physiologic effects from inhaled herbal dust particles, or from the vapors of alcohol extracts. If dusty or vaporous conditions are apparent in areas where herbs are weighed and packaged, improvements in ventilation and air filtration are the proper first response. If needed in addition to such engineering solutions, filtering masks may be used as personal protective equipment (PPE) - but OSHA allows this only if engineering and administrative solutions cannot be made adequate. (OSHA 1995)

Risk Control Strategies:
Avoid locations with chemical or mold odors, and with poor ventilation.

Install ventilation for indirect moxibustion or use infrared lamps.

Install ventilation and air filtration if dusty or vaporous conditions are apparent in areas where herbs are weighed and packaged.

Fall Injuries

Risks:
Liability for fall injuries.

Discussion:
The prevention of fall injuries begins with basic housekeeping practices. Clear all aisleways of clutter. Keep electric cords away from walkways. Secure rugs with anti-slip mats, double-sided carpet tape or tacks. If water is tracked in, an entry mat might help decrease slickness of the floor surface. Observe conditions, mop up water promptly, and place a warning sign on damp floors.

Ascertain that aisleways and entryways are well lit. Confirm that stairways have secure railings, and that the treads and risers are equally spaced and in good repair. Elevator access is preferable to stairs.

In cold climates, walkways outside the building should be maintained free of snow and ice. Delegation of this responsibility to the landlord in a lease transfers some (but not necessarily all) of the liability.

Risk Control Strategies:
Attend to housekeeping practices to keep aisleways clear of trip and slip hazards.

Assess aisleway lighting and stairway conditions for safety.

Clarify responsibility for snow removal and common area maintenance in the lease.

Obtain premises liability insurance policy.

Emergency Action & Fire Prevention Plans

Risks:
Lack of emergency preparedness; OSHA regulatory compliance.

Discussion:
What types of emergencies might occur at your practice? Emergency preparations can make a vital difference. Plan your responses to emergencies such as: fire, flood, hurricane, and earthquake. Develop responses for power failure, computer failure, and computer theft, as well. Medical emergency plans are discussed in Chapter 9.

OSHA requires that certain employers with **10** or more employees develop a written emergency action plan (29CFR1910.38(a)), and a written fire prevention plan (29CFR1910.38(b)). Employers with fewer employees may orally communicate these plans to employees. Acupuncturists are not among those employers generally mandated to have such plans. Nevertheless, comprehensive emergency action and fire prevention plans are an excellent idea. They define employee responses in emergency situations, and may contribute to preventing serious injuries. Examples of emergency action and fire prevention plans are located in Appendix A.

An OSHA <u>emergency action plan</u> must have at least the following elements:

* emergency evacuation procedures and routes, specified for different types of emergencies.

* procedures for employees with critical functions prior to evacuation.

* procedure to account for all employees after evacuation.

* employee rescue and medical duties (if any).

* means of reporting fires and other emergencies.

* name(s) or title(s) of plan administrator(s).

The employer must establish an alarm system to alert employees. For a small clinic, smoke detectors, carbon monoxide detectors and direct voice communication serve this purpose. While smoke detectors are essential safety devices, they can be inadvertently set off by indirect moxa smoke. See Chapter 15 for discussion of alternative forms of indirect moxa.

The employer must designate and train a sufficient number of individuals to assist in emergency evacuations. Employees must receive training when the plan is initiated, when it is changed, and when the employee's designated emergency actions change. As with all training, it is prudent for the employer to document the date, subject matter, and attendees at each training session. The written plan must be available for employee review. It is good practice to include a copy in the employee handbook, and to provide updated copies annually.

OSHA requires that all employers provide for employee safety in the event of fire. Oregon OSHA defines four options with respect to fire extinguishers. (OR.OSHA 1995) In Option A, portable fire extinguishers are provided in the workplace, but not intended for employee use. In case of fire, employees are to evacuate per an emergency action plan. This option reduces the employer's risk of employee injuries sustained fighting a fire, but it decreases small fire suppression capability. A fire prevention plan and extinguisher maintenance and testing are also required. In Option B, designated employees are allowed to use fire extinguishers. In addition to the requirements of Option A, the employer must annually train designated employees in extinguisher use. In Option C, all employees are allowed to use fire extinguishers. The employer must select extinguishers based on anticipated fire class (A,B,C,D); inspect, maintain and test the extinguishers; and distribute them so that no employee must travel more than 75 feet to reach an extinguisher. All employees must be trained in extinguisher use. In Option D, fire extinguishers are not provided and all employees must evacuate in case of fire. Emergency action and fire prevention plans are required. Options B and C appear the most sensible - fire extinguishers increase safety only if people are trained and allowed to use them. Contact your local fire department to inquire about training in fire extinguisher use.

The necessary elements of an OSHA <u>fire prevention plan</u> are:

> *   list of workplace fire hazards, potential ignition sources, storage and risk control procedures, and type of extinguisher needed for fire control.

* name or title of person responsible for maintaining fire prevention and control equipment.

* name or title of person responsible for control of flammable chemical hazards.

* housekeeping procedures to reduce accumulations of combustible waste materials.

* maintenance plan for heat producing equipment to reduce accidental fires.

Employers must alert employees to fire hazard exposures from workplace materials and processes. Employees must receive fire prevention plan training on initial assignment. The written plan must be available for employee review. It is good practice to include a copy in the employee handbook, and to provide updated copies annually.

Risk Control Strategies:
Plan your responses to the types of emergencies that might arise.

Write an emergency action plan and a fire prevention plan. Review annually, and include copies in the employee handbook and in orientation training.

Annually train all employees in their duties in response to major emergencies. Document this training.

Annually train designated (or all) employees in principles of fire extinguisher use, hazards of first stage fires, hands-on use of extinguishers, and when to evacuate. Document this training.

Conduct and document annual evacuation drills.

Post emergency evacuation procedures.

Mark exits and emergency exits with illuminated signs designed to stay lit in power outages.

Keep access to and opening of exit doors unobstructed from both inside and outside.

Clearly label doors that do not lead to exits, and that might be confused with exits (e.g. 'Storage Area').

Post exit directional signs in aisleways where exits are not visible.

Place a fire extinguisher sign above extinguishers, to facilitate location in emergencies. Maintain unobstructed access.

Document periodic inspection, testing and maintenance of fire extinguishers, smoke detectors, carbon monoxide detectors, and/or automatic sprinkler systems. Install where appropriate.

Some localities require a fire marshall's inspection and approval prior to opening an office. Check with your local authorities.

OSHA Chemical Hazard Communication Standard

Risks:
Accidental poisoning or chemical injury; fire hazard; OSHA regulatory compliance.

Discussion:
The OSHA Hazard Communication Standard (HCS) (29CFR1910.1200) applies to all employers. The intent of the HCS

is to inform exposed employees about the identities and dangers of all hazardous chemicals in the workplace, and about related protective measures. See Appendix B for the full regulatory text.

A chemical hazard communication program is required. A sample program is in Appendix A. The program is comprised of:

* written hazard communication program.

* container labeling.

* file of Material Safety Data Sheets (MSDS).

* documented employee training.

What are the elements of a written hazard communication program? The program must state how you will meet labeling, MSDS and employee training requirements. It also must include a list of hazardous chemicals in your workplace. It must describe how you will inform employees of hazards they might be exposed to in non-routine tasks. The written program can be used as part of your employee training materials.

What substances in acupuncture offices are considered hazardous? Alcohol, sterilants and disinfectants, iodine and bleach are commonly present and hazardous. Items such as 'white out', while potentially toxic, are present in small enough quantities to pose insignificant risk, and need not be included in a hazardous chemicals list. The determination and evaluation of chemical hazards is a formal process best left to manufacturers, whose responsibilities include publishing MSDS's for their products.

The employer is responsible for labeling each hazardous chemical container in the workplace. When hazardous chemicals are decanted from their original containers into secondary containers, those secondary containers must also be labeled. Labels must indicate the common or chemical name, and must summarize the hazards associated with its use. The inclusion of precautions is voluntary. For example, an alcohol disinfectant container might be labeled:

DANGER
70% ISOPROPYL ALCOHOL
POISON HAZARD, FIRE HAZARD
KEEP CONTAINER CLOSED & AWAY FROM FLAME
FOR EXTERNAL USE ONLY

Labels must be legible and in English, although additional languages may be added. The name of the substance must be the same as printed on the related MSDS.

Employers must keep a current file of MSDS's for each hazardous chemical in the workplace. These can be obtained from manufacturers and suppliers, and can also be retrieved from several Internet sites. (See Resources) MSDS's must be filed and retained for at least **30** years. (29CFR1910.20(d)(1)(ii)). Periodically the MSDS files must be updated to reflect any new hazard information that may have been developed. Employees must have ready access to the MSDS file. Employees must be trained to recognize the hazards and take the protective measures indicated in the MSDS's. The MSDS's must be available in English, although the inclusion of additional languages is optional.

A sample MSDS is in Appendix A. An MSDS must contain at least the following information:

* chemical and common name of the hazardous substance.

* physical and chemical characteristics of the hazardous substance.

* physical hazards (fire explosion, reactivity).

* health hazards, including signs and symptoms of exposure.

* primary routes of entry.

* OSHA exposure limits, where available.

* whether the chemical is a listed carcinogen.

* precautions for safe handling and use.

* engineering, work practice and personal protective equipment (PPE) risk control measures.

* emergency and first aid procedures.

* MSDS preparation date or update.

* contact information for preparer of the MSDS.

Employees must be trained prior to initial use of hazardous chemicals. Periodic re-training (e.g annually, and whenever new hazardous chemicals enter the workplace) is recommended. A training program must instruct employees in:

* location and identity of hazardous chemicals.

* requirements of the Hazard Communication Rules.

* availability and location of your written program.

* availability and location of hazardous chemicals list.

* availability and location of the MSDS file.

* physical and health hazards of the chemicals.

* labeling system used.

* chemical hazard protective practices in your workplace.

* type, limitations, demonstrated use & location of PPE.

* recognition of dangerous release of chemicals.

* emergency and first aid procedures.

The training program must include an opportunity for employee questions to be answered. Assessments of effectiveness, such as a test and employee feedback, are valuable components which can lead to improvements in the training program. It is good practice to document attendance. See Resources for training materials.

Contractors working on-site must be informed of chemical hazards, controls, and location of the MSDS file.

Risk Control Strategies:
Develop a written chemical hazard communication program. Review at least annually and update as needed.

Label all containers of hazardous chemicals with the chemical or common name and a summary of hazards and safety practices.

Inventory hazardous chemicals, their maximum quantities and storage locations.

Obtain and file chemical MSDS's. Update the MSDS file at least annually, and whenever new chemical hazards enter the workplace.

Maintain MSDS files for at least **30** years.

Develop a chemical hazard training program. Deliver training to all current employees, and to new employees prior to their use of any hazardous chemicals.

Document training attendance and effectiveness evaluations.

Repeat training at least annually, and whenever new chemical hazards enter the workplace.

CHAPTER 5

EMPLOYERS & EMPLOYEES

In the context of Employers & Employees we introduce employer's basic duties; hiring & firing; policies & procedures; the provision of optimal ergonomic work conditions; and implications of accepting the conditions of work.

Employer's Basic Duties

Risks:
Basic regulatory and tax compliance.

Discussion:
In addition to licenses and permits for the operation of a business, employers must register with local, state and federal governments to arrange for payment of payroll taxes and workers compensation insurance taxes. Tax statements are usually due quarterly, and should be filed timely. Many businesses find it convenient to either use a computer program or a payroll service to calculate salary withholdings and net wages.

OSHA requires employers to permanently post the 'OSHA Job Safety & Health Poster' - an informational page about job safety and OSHA - in a location where all employees can access it. An ADA poster required if there are **15** or more employees. States may also have required postings, such as minimum wage notices. These are usually supplied with business registration materials received from the state's business registry.

Employers with **10** or more employees must post the OSHA 200 form (an occupational injury and illness log) throughout the month of February. The OSHA 101, a supplemental companion form, must also be maintained. OHSA is considering replacing these forms in 1999 with OSHA 300 and 301 forms respectively. Colleges are usually exempted from these requirements.

Record bloodborne pathogen exposure incidents on the OSHA 200 form, and any injuries where the recommended medical treatment goes beyond first aid. If an exposure incident results in seroconversion, that diagnosis should not be recorded on the form, because it is confidential information. Instead, enter the causal injury (e.g. needlestick injury). The OSHA 200 form must be retained for at least **5** years.

The employer has a duty to maintain a safe and sanitary workplace. The standards of performance are defined through OSHA regulations detailed in Chapters 4 and 6.

Risk Control Strategies:
Obtain and post all necessary licenses, permits and posters.

Remit paychecks and quarterly payroll taxes on time.

Maintain safe and sanitary work conditions as defined by OSHA.

Hiring & Firing

Risks:
Liability for employment practices.

Discussion:
Employers have a duty to hire qualified personnel. Failure to do so may engender liability for negligent hiring and supervision. It is prudent to inquire about the existence of previous felonies, crimes, professional disciplinary proceedings, or malpractice claims, which might reflect on the applicant's job performance. It is incumbent on the employer to set training prerequisites, verify applicant training and credentials, and verify personal and professional references. Performance tests should be uniformly given to all applicants if given to any, and should be germane to the job description. Failure to exercise due care in hiring increases the employer's liability for untoward actions of the employee.

Employers have a duty to employ without regard to a variety of extraneous individual qualities. This is mandated by the Civil Rights Act of 1964 and 1991, the Age Discrimination In Employment Act of 1967, the Rehabilitation Act of 1973, and the Pregnancy Discrimination Act of 1978. The Equal Employment Opportunities Commission monitors violations of several of these acts. (Arthur 1995) Avoid interview questions about age, race, gender, sexual orientation, marital status, daycare plans, height and weight, credit history, religious affiliation and practices, political beliefs, national origin, illness history and disabilities. A job offer should be predicated on meeting qualifications defined in a written job description. The job description is the basis for hiring, performance evaluation, discipline, reward, promotion, demotion, and termination actions. Do not overlook mention of interpersonal skills and qualities in a job description, as these are necessary attributes of functional employees.

Employers with **15** or more employees are compelled by the ADA to equitably consider applicants with disabilities for employment, whenever job performance and safety are not compromised and reasonable accommodation can be made. (USDOJ 1992) Note that while alcoholism is a disability as defined by the ADA, it may significantly compromise job performance, safety and judgment.

The Immigration Reform And Control Act of 1986 requires employers to verify new employees' citizenship status within 3 days of hiring, and then file federal Form I-9. A U.S. passport establishes identity and employability, as does the combination of a U.S. driver's license and social security card. It is legal to hire non-citizens who have a visa or naturalization documents that permit them to be employed.

It is worthy to note that the Equal Pay Act of 1963 mandates equal pay for men and women in the same job classification, with individual differences allowed based on educational attainment, experience and seniority.

By conducting periodic performance evaluations, the employer can clearly communicate and document how expectations have been met, exceeded or unmet. Evaluations are an opportunity to reward fine performance and delineate improvements in substandard performance. Written evaluations substantiate the merit of promotion, demotion, or termination actions.

Employers are well advised to have a written employee termination policy, in this day of wrongful termination actions against employers. In particular, attend to adequate notice provisions and consistent procedures to determine the existence of grounds for termination.

When providing a reference for a former employee, the former employer should speak or write with discretion to avoid misleading the potential employer, and to avoid defaming the reputation of the former employee. Any negative information should be substantiated in the employees's file to avoid liability for slander or libel.

Once a new employee has been hired, complete orientation and training before that employee assumes clinical responsibilities. Employers should provide emergency action plan, fire prevention plan, chemical hazard communication and bloodborne pathogen training. The first HBV vaccination should be made available after completion of bloodborne pathogen training. (See Chapter 6.) Training prior to clinical placement optimally protects employer, employee and patients.

Employers are encouraged to consult textual resources on employment and the law (Arthur 1995; Dickson 1995), and state Employment Departments, for more information.

Risk Control Strategies:
Base hiring on qualifications defined in a written job description.

Avoid interview questions about extraneous personal attributes.

Focus interview questions on abilities to perform job tasks, and assess the personality traits that relate to organizational function.

Contact references and verify training and credentials.

Accommodate disabilities whenever job performance and safety are not compromised and the accommodation is readily achievable.

Provide and file copies of employee performance evaluations.

If contemplating termination, document all performance based reasons, notices to the employee, actions taken to remedy the situation, and circumstances justifying termination.

When providing a reference for a former employee, speak or write with discretion to avoid misleading the potential employer or defaming the reputation of the former employee.

Provide and document training for new employees before they assume clinical responsibilities.

Policies & Procedures

Risks:
Liabilities related to lack of documented exposition of policies and standard operating procedures.

Discussion:
An Employee Handbook (EH) informs employees about policies and operating procedures, and communicates mutual expectations. It should address employment policies including hiring policies, dispute resolution, performance evaluation, discipline and termination procedures, attendance standards, pay policies, benefits, vacations, leaves, and work rules. State any appearance codes, sexual harassment policies and drug policies. Safety procedures and expected safe work practices should also be well elucidated, for the protection of patients, employees and the employer.

The EH can be interpreted as a contract, and must be drafted with care. Employers are referred to a textual resource with carefully worded policy statements that are designed to be used verbatim. (Harper Business 1990)

Risk Control Strategies:
Develop an Employee Handbook which defines office policies and standard operating procedures.

Include emergency action plan, fire prevention plan, chemical hazards communication program, and bloodborne pathogens exposure control plan information.

Provision Of Optimal Ergonomic Work Conditions

Risks:
Employee discomfort, injury, and lost productivity.
Increased workers compensation insurance costs.

Discussion:
Ergonomics is about designing work to fit the body. If you employ others in your practice (receptionists, clinical assistants, etc.), provide optimal ergonomic work conditions for them. Preventing work-related injuries improves productivity and keeps your workers compensation insurance payments low. Occupational repetitive stress injuries (RSI's) cost U.S. employers roughly $20 billion in 1993, just in workers compensation claims. Indirect costs were estimated at $100 billion. (OSHA 1997) OSHA is considering (but has not enacted) comprehensive ergonomic standards.

In assessing secretarial and treatment workstations, consider these primarily ergonomic components of safety:

Lighting: Is lighting sufficient to provide easy visibility with neither eyestrain nor glare? Consider full spectrum lighting (i.e. color balanced as found in natural sunlight), which also enhances the ability to judge colors in TOM diagnosis.

Seating: Are chairs comfortable and adjustable to the proportions of the actual users? Ergonomically suitable chairs are designed with many adjustable features to allow for proper seated posture, reducing bodily strain and fatigue. The seated person's feet should be able to rest on the ground, and the lumbar spine should be well supported. No single make of chair is ergonomically correct for all users, even though the chair may be advertised as having an ergonomic design. The key criterion is fitness to the proportions of the actual user(s).

Secretarial Equipment Positioning: Are keyboards placed at a level to minimize wrist strain? Are desk edges in front of the keyboard cushioned? RSI's such as carpal tunnel syndrome are an increasingly common and expensive category of office injury. The problem can result from chronic forearm muscle tension caused by improper equipment positioning. Improperly placed computer monitors are of concern. Ideally they should be placed directly over the center of the keyboard, such that one can shift between viewing the screen and the keyboard with no head movement and minimal refocus. Also consider the effects of the telephone receiver on the position of the neck. If an employee spends much time on the phone, install a headset receiver.

Treatment Table Positioning: Are treatment tables at a height that facilitate work without bending over or reaching uncomfortably? Are tables sturdy and wide enough to hold and safely reposition very heavy patients? Is there a sturdy one-step stool to help patients up and down? Are tables positioned to afford access to both sides and to the head or foot? Optimize ability to see and minimize distances to reach, so that you may perform technical interventions with ease, accuracy, dexterity and control.

Risk Control Strategies:
Assess ergonomic factors and correct as needed for lighting, seating, and equipment positioning.

Accepting Conditions Of Work

Risks:
Injury to patients and employees arising from unsafe conditions.

Discussion:
At all times and regardless of being in the employ of any other party, acupuncturists are accountable and legally liable for unsafe practices. In the event of an adverse outcome, the acupuncturist's independent judgment (and license to practice) will be called into question, even if the unsafe conditions were created by the employer.

Assess the clinical setting for safety and standards of practice. If you believe conditions of work present a clear and present danger, or are remarkably sub-standard, do not proceed with treatments until those conditions are corrected.

If you notice sub-optimal clinical conditions for acupuncture while in the employ of another person, institution or agency, submit written requests for improvements (and save copies of that correspondence). You will have acted conscientiously to improve patient care and to marginally decrease personal liability.

Risk Control Strategies:
Do not proceed with work if conditions are unsafe.

Advise employer in writing regarding sub-standard conditions.

Obtain professional liability insurance.

CHAPTER 6

BLOODBORNE PATHOGENS

The OSHA Bloodborne Pathogens Standard requires employers to develop and implement an Exposure Control Plan based on an employee exposure risk determination. The employer must define methods of compliance involving specific engineering and work practice risk controls, informed by the concept of Universal Precautions. An HBV vaccination program and a post-exposure evaluation and follow-up plan are required. There are hazard labeling, employee training, and recordkeeping requirements as well.

OSHA Bloodborne Pathogens Standard

Overview:

The Bloodborne Pathogens Standard (BPS), 29CFR1910.1030, was enacted to protect employees from illnesses transmitted by contact with blood or 'other potentially infectious material' (OPIM). Hepatitis B virus (HBV), Hepatitis C virus (HCV) and the AIDS virus (HIV) are noteworthy among pathogens capable of causing serious illness and death. The hazards are significant - about 8,700 U.S. healthcare workers per year contract Hepatitis B through occupational exposures. (OSHA 1996) Blood, vaginal secretions, semen, amniotic fluid, cerebrospinal fluid, synovial fluid, and any visibly bloody body fluids are potentially infectious. Readers are advised to review a detailed account of infection risks and symptoms, such as MMWR 1989.

For a bloodborne infection to be transmitted, infectious blood or OPIM from a source person must contact the blood or mucous membranes of another person. Intact skin is a protective barrier, but cuts, abrasions and small cracks in the skin can allow pathogens to enter. Breaks in the skin are particularly common on the hands and around the fingernails.

The BPS applies to every occupation with the potential for blood exposure. It applies to all acupuncturists with clinical employees or other employees who might be at risk in the course of their duties (such as an assistant who cleans contaminated equipment, or a designated first aid provider). It applies to acupuncture college clinics with clinical employees, although it does not apply to students (except those students who are also clinical employees). Self-employed acupuncturists in solo practice or partnership, who have no clinical or other employees at risk, and who have not elected for workers compensation coverage for themselves, are not subject to the BPS. However, if an acupuncturist incorporates her business, then she is a corporate employee, and subject to the BPS.

Whether or not the BPS must be applied to your work situation, compliance with its requirements provides such significant risk control that it is difficult to defend practicing at a lower standard.

Prevention and safety are mandatory from a moral perspective. The full text of the BPS is in Appendix C.

Exposure Control Plan

Discussion:
The BPS requires employers to develop and implement a written Exposure Control Plan (ECP), which must be reviewed and updated

at least annually and whenever new procedures affect work exposure. The ECP must be accessible to employees. Examples of an ECP, and several related forms, are in Appendix A.

Elements of an ECP include: employee exposure risk determination; methods of compliance; HBV vaccination program; post-exposure evaluation and follow-up plans; communication of hazards to employees; and recordkeeping requirements.

Your ECP must designate an implementation schedule. Note immediate implementation, as BPS requirements have been in effect since 1992. We will proceed to discuss ECP components.

Exposure Risk Determination

Discussion:
The employer must define two groups of job classifications: those in which all of the employees in the job classification have exposure risks, and those in which only some of the employees in the job classification have exposure risk. For this latter group, the specific tasks with exposure risk must be listed.

For a small acupuncture practice, 'acupuncturist' might be the only job classification with exposure risk. Specific hazards are related to needling, cupping, coining, acupressure, equipment decontamination, housekeeping, regulated waste disposal and the provision of first aid. Refer to additional material in Chapters 9, 13, 14, 16, 17 and 19 for more information on those hazards. If employees other than acupuncturists clean blood or OPIM contaminated equipment or environmental surfaces, or are designated as first aid providers, then they would also be identified as employees at risk of exposure. Does emptying clinic garbage cans, or handling used linens (not visibly contaminated with blood), constitute risk of exposure? That is left to the judgment of the employer. (OSHA 1994)

Methods Of Compliance

Discussion:
After employees at risk and specific tasks with risk have been identified, your ECP then defines methods of compliance to eliminate or minimize employee bloodborne pathogen exposures. Methods of compliance include using the concept of universal precautions, and implementing a range of engineering and work practice controls. Let us examine these in greater detail.

Universal Precautions

Discussion:
'Universal Precautions' is a BPS-required approach to infection control. It is based on the presumption that all blood and OPIM are infectious (since we do not know the infectious status of most people's blood). By this standard, every potential exposure must be avoided, and the procedures used for every patient must be adequate for protection if their blood were in fact infectious.

This does not imply that providers are forbidden to use higher levels of diligence and precaution in cases where the patient's infection risk is confirmed by biomedical diagnosis. According to the Centers for Disease Control & Prevention (CDC):

> Exceptional circumstances that require noncritical items to be either dedicated to one patient or patient cohort, or

subjected to low-level disinfection between patient uses, are those involving: Patients infected or colonized with vancomycin-resistant enterococci or other drug-resistant microorganisms judged by the infection control program, based on current state, regional, or national recommendations, to be of special or clinical or epidemiologic significance, or: Patients infected with highly virulent microorganisms, e.g., viruses causing hemorrhagic fever (such as Ebola or Lassa). (CDC 1997)

A protocol for high risk patients is described in NAF 1997.

Engineering Controls

Discussion:
Engineering controls reduce exposure risk by removing a hazard or isolating the worker from exposure. The use of puncture-resistant red plastic sharps containers for immediate containment of contaminated needles are the most significant engineering control in an acupuncture practice. Sharps containers must be located in close proximity to areas of needle use. They must be attached to a wall or counter surface to prevent being knocked over. Sharps containers must be replaced before becoming over-filled, and must be disposed of as regulated medical waste in compliance with local, state and federal regulations.

Work Practice Controls

Discussion:
Work practice controls define the way tasks are to be performed to reduce exposure risk. Work practice controls include handwashing

practices; general work procedures and specific work procedures. Personal protective equipment and housekeeping protocols are important extensions of work practices. We will examine these topics in order.

Handwashing

Discussion:
Handwashing is the simplest, most cost effective and most important work practice in preventing the transmission of bloodborne pathogens. (CDC 1985) Adherence to required handwashing practices is an essential component of compliance.

The BPS requires that employers provide handwashing facilities, and that those facilities be close to the work area. The regulations also require that hands be washed with soap and running water immediately after removal of gloves or other PPE. Body areas contacting blood or OPIM must be washed (or in the case of eyes or mucous membranes, rinsed) immediately after exposure.

Washing with plain soap effectively reduces transient microorganisms, while the deeper resident microorganisms are more effectively killed or inhibited by anti-microbial soaps. Liquid soap dispensers may become contaminated, and should be replaced when empty. (CDC 1985) In the absence of anti-microbial soap, use a germicidal towelette (e.g. Hibistat®), an alcohol foam (e.g. AlCare®), or a liquid hand sanitizer (e.g. Purell®).

Acupuncturists should wash hands before needle insertion, between each patient contact, after removing gloves, and immediately after any blood or OPIM exposure. Prior to resuming patient care, hands should be washed after using the toilet, and after touching nasal passages or blowing the nose.

The following is a protocol for handwashing and hand care:

- * Keep fingernails closely trimmed.

- * Remove rings that protrude or do not have smooth surfaces.

- * Use paper towel to turn faucets on. Do not use this towel to dry hands.

- * Use disinfectant soap supplied in leaflets or by disposable pump dispenser. Do not touch pump spout.

- * Apply soap to wet hands; wash for 10-15 seconds, scrubbing finger tips, between fingers, and palms up to the wrists. Rinse.

- * Dry with single use towel or hot air dryer.

- * Use paper towel to turn faucets off, without letting hands contact faucet handles.

- * Dispose used towels in plastic bag lined trash can.

To avoid patient and employee injury from scalding hot water, adjust the hot water heater thermostat to 125-130°F.

For handwashing resources, refer to USDHHS 1988; NAF 1997.

General Work Procedures

Discussion:
In areas where occupational exposure to blood or OPIM may occur, general work procedures to control risk include not allowing eating, drinking, smoking, cosmetic or lip balm application or contact lens handling. Food and drink must not be stored in refrigerators or other areas where blood or OPIM are present.

Procedures involving blood or OPIM must be performed in ways that prevent splashing, spraying or spattering.

Specific Work Procedures

Discussion:
For each task with risk of exposure, the employer must define safe work protocols required of employees. Refer to Chapters 13, 14, 16, 17 & 19 for protocols related to environmental and equipment decontamination, needling, cupping, coining and acupressure.

Personal Protective Equipment

Discussion:
Personal protective equipment (PPE) is used to control exposure risks that remain after the implementation of engineering controls and other safer work practices. PPE includes gloves, lab coats, resuscitation barriers, face shields and eye protection. Your ECP should identify tasks that require PPE, and type of PPE to be used.

Employers must provide PPE in fitting sizes, at no cost, to all employees at risk of exposure. Employers must <u>require</u> the use of

PPE when it is the appropriate exposure control measure, which is to say whenever an occupational exposure may be reasonably anticipated to occur. Employers are accountable for the correct use, cleaning, replacement and disposal of PPE.

Non-sterile latex (or vinyl) exam gloves, and rubber utility gloves are appropriate PPE for common exposure-prone tasks in an acupuncture practice. Refer to Chapters 9, 16 and 21 for additional PPE recommendations related to first aid, cupping and lasers.

Latex exam gloves are disposables intended for single use in ordinary patient care procedures. Their routine use during needle removal is discussed in Chapter 14. They must be removed before leaving the work area, and whenever they become contaminated, punctured or torn. Rings may need to be removed before donning gloves to prevent tearing the gloves. Petroleum based hand lotions should not be used because petroleum products degrade latex, first making it more porous and then melting it. Petroleum based massage oils and coining lubricants also should be avoided when working gloved, for the same reason. Latex also degrades in contact with some vegetable oils and their components, including castor oil, flaxseed oil, linoleic acid, and to a lesser extent, oleic acid. Palmitic acid does not affect latex. Latex gloves should not be washed, as surfactants degrade latex. Water-based lotions and lubricants and glycerin-based products do not degrade latex. (CDC 1997a; CDC 1997b)

While latex gloves provide barrier protection for the hands, they introduce a risk of latex allergy reactions in the user and in patients who are touched by latex gloves. Inquire about latex allergy on your patient medical history form. Symptoms include skin rashes, hives, itching, sinus or eye symptoms, asthma, and (rarely) shock. Un-powdered low-protein latex gloves, and vinyl gloves, tend to be less allergenic. (NIOSH 1997) Handwashing after glove removal decreases exposure to the latex proteins. Vinyl gloves may be substituted for latex, but many users find lesser dexterity in vinyl gloves. Hypo-allergenic gloves must be made available to employees allergic to latex gloves.

Instruct employees in proper glove removal. The tip of one glove cuff is pinched and pulled toward the fingers, turning the glove inside out. The removed glove is held in the palm of the other gloved hand while the procedure is repeated. This encases the first glove inside the second inverted glove, and minimizes contact with contaminated glove surfaces. Dispose of used gloves (as contaminated waste, unless covered with blood) in a trash can lined with a plastic bag.

Rubber utility gloves may be reused after decontamination if not damaged. They are suitable for office housekeeping, decontamination chores, and heavier cleaning duties.

If lab coats are worn as PPE, they must be supplied and laundered at the employer's expense, and may not be taken home for cleaning by employees. If lab coats are worn as a professional costume with no reasonable need for or intent of PPE function (and this is noted in your ECP), then such restrictions do not apply.

Housekeeping

Discussion:
The BPS requires the employer to maintain a clean and sanitary facility. Your ECP will define a written cleaning schedule, and will list the methods of decontamination and tasks to be performed.

Contaminated work surfaces must be cleaned with a tuberculocidal disinfectant as soon as feasible. Potentially contaminated work surfaces must be routinely cleaned. Trash receptacles must be decontaminated on a scheduled basis, and whenever obviously contaminated. Clean horizontal surfaces in patient care areas on a regular basis.

Methods of decontamination must be stated. Refer to Chapter 13 for a discussion of decontamination protocols. Rubber utility gloves are necessary PPE for decontamination chores.

Contaminated laundry is defined as being soiled with blood or OPIM, or as laundry which may contain sharps. The cleaning facility where these will be laundered must be identified in the ECP. Contaminated laundry may not be taken home for laundering. Handle it as little as possible, and place it in labeled containers.

Your ECP will define procedures for removing broken glass. Broken glass must never be directly handled, even with gloved hands. It is safer to use a dust pan, brush and tongs.

Under the rubric of Housekeeping, your ECP will address the handling, containment and disposal of regulated waste and contaminated waste. <u>Regulated waste</u> is a category of biohazardous medical waste requiring very special storage, labeling and disposal. Regulated waste includes used needles (sharps), as well as items so saturated with blood or OPIM that if compressed they would leak. Used needles are immediately disposed of in red sharps containers and later transferred to a regulated waste disposal company. (Refer to Chapter 14.) All other non-sharp regulated waste must be sealed in red plastic bags ('red bagged') for removal by a regulated waste disposal company. Readers are advised to consult state and local agencies to determine additional requirements for regulated waste disposal.

Contaminated waste includes materials that may have blood or OPIM present, but in not in a quantity sufficient to shed or release it when the waste is being handled. Used cotton balls (even with several drops of blood on them), used bandages, and used sanitary napkins are all defined as contaminated waste, as long as they do not meet the definition of regulated waste. Sealing contaminated waste in plastic trash bags is sufficient containment. Contaminated waste may be placed in the regular trash stream. Rubber utility gloves are appropriate PPE for trash handling. If there is any doubt as to whether an article is regulated or contaminated waste, it is safer to consider it regulated waste.

Hepatitis B Vaccination

Discussion:
For all employees with occupational bloodborne pathogen exposure risk, employers are required to make available a series of three HBV vaccinations, at no cost to employees. The vaccination must be made available within **10** working days of initial assignment, and after completion of bloodborne pathogen training. Completion of the first immunization prior to the initial clinical assignment increases the margin of safety for employees and employer. Each employee's HBV vaccination status and each vaccination date must be recorded in their employee medical record. Employees who decline the vaccination must sign a special 'declination form'. (See Appendix A) Employees declining the vaccinations may later opt to receive them, without charge.

The vaccine contains an HBV surface antigen which has been produced by genetically re-engineered yeast. It is not a live virus vaccine and cannot transmit hepatitis. It is also not a human or animal blood product, and cannot transmit HIV. The vaccine is approximately 96% effective in preventing HBV infection. It provides lesser but significant protection when first administered promptly after a needlestick injury. (MMWR 1989) The series of vaccinations costs employers about $200.00 per employee.

Employees who have earlier completed the immunization series, or who on blood testing show sufficient immunity gained from prior exposure to HBV, are exempted from vaccination and should sign the declination form. Exemptions are also made for employees with medical contraindications documented by a physician.

Exposure Evaluation & Follow-Up Plan

Discussion:
When there is unprotected occupational contact with blood or OPIM, an exposure incident has occurred. It may involve an accidental needlestick with a contaminated needle, or direct hand contact with blood or OPIM. There might be blood or OPIM contact to the eyes or mouth, perhaps during a first aid procedure. The employer must have a written plan defining employee response, and providing for evaluation and care of employees involved in exposure incidents.

The employee must immediately wash the exposed area (or rinse eyes or mucous membranes if they were exposed to blood or OPIM), and then promptly report the incident to the employer. The employer must then refer the employee to a healthcare provider (designated in the plan) for medical evaluation, treatment and follow-up. Time is of the essence where HIV infection is a possibility, as chemoprophylaxis should be initiated within 1-2 hours of exposure. (CD Summary 1996)

The employer must transmit the following documents to the healthcare provider:

* Copy of the BPS.

* Description of the employee's exposure-related job duties.

* Report of the specific exposure incident & route of exposure ('Incident Report').

* HBV vaccination status and any other relevant employee medical records.

Relatively few healthcare providers continually stock HBV vaccine and HIV chemoprophylaxis supplies. In the immediate aftermath of an exposure incident, they will evaluate the need for such interventions, and if necessary direct the employee to the nearest hospital emergency room where such medications are available.

The healthcare provider's evaluation and follow-up must include:

* Statement of how exposure occurred & route of exposure.

* Identity of the source individual (unless prohibited by state law).

* Test of source individual's blood to determine infectivity (consent is usually required). If known infective for HIV or HBV, testing need not be repeated.

* Test of employee's blood to determine HIV and HBV serologic status (consent is required).

* Provide employee with source individual's test results, and advise on regulations limiting disclosure of source identity and infectious status.

* Provide post-exposure treatment and counseling following U.S. Public Health Service guidelines.

* Report ('Written Opinion') to employer within 15 days, limited to (a) statement that employee has been informed of test results and advised of any need for more treatment or follow-up; and (b) whether vaccine has been administered. (All other medical information is protected by patient/provider confidentiality.)

The employer must then provide the employee with a copy of the written opinion report within **15** days, and place a copy in the employee's medical record.

If an employee refuses baseline HIV testing after an exposure incident, but accepts HBV testing, the blood sample must be preserved 90 days. Should the employee elect to have the HIV test within that time, it must be done.

All exposure incident evaluation, treatment and follow-up costs are required to be borne by the employer. The employer additionally must evaluate the circumstances of an exposure incident and consider risk control measures to prevent reoccurrences.

Biohazard Labeling

Discussion:

Regulated waste containers (such as sharps containers) must have a fluorescent orange or red-orange label with the biohazard symbol and have the word BIOHAZARD on them, and/or be red in color. Red plastic waste bags do not require the biohazard label, but employees must be trained to know red bags contain regulated waste. The biohazard symbol is shown in *Figure 6.1*.

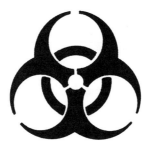

Figure 6.1 - Biohazard Symbol

Bloodborne Pathogen Hazard Training

Discussion:

The employer must provide and document bloodborne pathogen training for every at-risk employee, at no cost to the employee. That training must be provided on work time, at the time of initial assignment. The training must be repeated at least once per year, or whenever tasks are modified in a way that affects exposure risk. See Recordkeeping for training documentation requirements.

Training programs must include:

* How to obtain a copy of the BPS and the employer's ECP, and a summary of their contents.

* Epidemiology, symptoms & routes of transmission of major bloodborne pathogens.

* Explanation of tasks with exposure risks.

* Explanation of uses & limits of site-specific engineering & work practice controls.

* PPE location, types, proper use, removal, decontamination & disposal.

* HBV Vaccination information.

* How to respond to exposure incidents & the nature of post-exposure evaluation and care.

* Information about warning labels, color coding and hazard signs.

* Emergency response procedures and whom to contact in an emergency.

* Questions and answer session.

Trainers must be knowledgeable and able to document their own education in bloodborne pathogens. Videos may be used for most of the training, but a live question and answer session and site-specific training must be provided. Training should not just cover the bases - it must be effective. OSHA evaluates the adequacy of training by employee performance. A written test administered after training documents employee comprehension. It is good practice to keep test results on file. See Resources for training video suppliers.

Recordkeeping

Discussion:
The BPS mandates that employers keep training records and employee medical records.

Employers must keep <u>training records</u> for at least **3** years. The training record must contain:

* Training dates.

* Summary of the training program.

* Trainer's name & qualifications.

* Names & job titles of trainees.

Employee <u>medical records</u> must be kept confidential. They are to be maintained for **30** years beyond the duration of employment. In the sale of a practice, transfer the records to the new owner. If a practice closes without a successor, the employer must notify the director of National Institute for Occupational Safety and Health (NIOSH) for directions on employee records disposition. NIOSH and OSHA have a right to access employee medical and training records without employee authorization. Employees have a right to obtain copies of their own medical and training records.

The medical record must include:

* Name & social security number (SSN) of employee.

* HBV vaccination status, vaccination dates, and records related to ability to receive vaccinations.

* Results of pre-exposure and post-exposure tests, evaluations and follow-up procedures.

* Copy of information provided to the evaluating medical provider.

* Medical provider written opinion report to employer.

To protect confidentiality and to increase speed of post-exposure medical provider access to an employee's medical record, many employers opt to store employee medical records at the designated post-exposure medical provider's office. In this instance, the employer should keep a duplicate 'administrative record' for each employee, which would not include results of pre-exposure and post-exposure tests, evaluations and follow-up procedures. Nothing in the duplicate record should indicate an employee's HIV or HBV infectious status. The employer must document where the full medical records are located.

An important reminder: federal OSHA regulations are often modified by state OSHA agency regulations. If your state has an OSHA agency, then contact them for BPS and all other OSHA regulatory compliance guidance. OSHA encourages such proactive compliance efforts, and provides employers with free consultation services.

The BPS places many obligations on employers, and it is easy to consider those obligations to be external burdens. But thoughtful employers recognize a moral obligation to protect employees. The BPS regulations are a formal means of helping your practice fulfill the internal obligation to assess and manage serious risks. Following an Exposure Control Plan will save lives - and one of those lives may be your own.

Risk Control Strategies:
If your practice has any bloodborne pathogen risks, develop and implement all aspects of the Bloodborne Pathogens Exposure Control Plan, whether you have employees or not.

CHAPTER 7

RECORDS & BILLING

Arising from the context of Records & Billing are risks associated with medical record contents; record confidentiality & release; and record retention & destruction. Treatment limits & billing limits; ethical billing practices; and collection practices are then presented. The chapter closes with review of procedure codes; and diagnostic codes as related to scope of practice.

Medical Record Contents

Risks:
Presumption of negligence, and possible violation of state and federal mandates to document care.

Discussion:
Medical records are both clinical and legal documents. In statutory law, and more broadly in common law, the failure to adequately document patient care can be deemed evidence of negligence. Medical record contents are defined by laws and regulations, and also by professional, accrediting and institutional standards. To participate in Medicare programs, the federal Department of Health & Human Services requires the record be sufficient to identify the patient, justify the diagnosis and treatment, and to document the results. Detailed professional guidelines are published by the American Health Information Management Association, and by Joint Commission on Accreditation of Healthcare Organizations. (AHIMA 1992; JCAHO 1995) These resources present a standard

for medical records practices by acupuncturists. While the specifics of diagnosis and treatment are unique to TOM, the context and form of medical records are generic to American medicine.

Medical records should be complete in several regards. From a legal perspective, *if an action, observation or conversation isn't charted, it is assumed not to have happened.* Malpractice attorneys bemoan that medical providers spend years developing advanced diagnostic and therapeutic reasoning processes, but then often fail to provide evidence of same in their chart notes.

A complete record provides:

* patient identification information.

* prior medical history.

* dated consent forms or record of consent process.

* evidence of assessment of the patient's condition.

* plan of care.

* date, time, and descriptive record of each treatment.

* progress notes, observations and clinical findings.

* discharge summary with final diagnosis, prognosis.

* authorship of all medical record entries.

Completeness vies with discretion in the matter of what to write, and what not to write, in the patient's chart. Personal and derogatory assessments of the patient's character have no place in the medical record ('Chronic complainer late for appointment again.'). Discretion weighs against including personal confidences the patient has shared with the provider, unless this material is pertinent to psychologic or medical therapy. The diagnoses applied in charting and billing are of critical importance with regard to scope of practice and social repercussions. Refer to Diagnostic Codes & Scope Of Practice, below.

Chart notes are written in a formalized style which tends to be terse in description and cautionary in conclusion, while nevertheless conveying the most essential information. The style is learned by reading and analyzing examples of fine medical charting, and then it is refined through peer review critiques of charting.

SOAP notes are a common nursing format for charting. SOAP is an acronym for Subjective, Objective, Assessment and Plan, the section titles used in recording each patient visit. Record of the initial visit is relatively extensive, and it is drawn on by reference to generate concise reports of subsequent visits. (Seidel et al 1991)

In the Subjective section, the patient's experience and perceptions of their problem are recorded. This information includes patient description of each complaint with its history, progression, symptom location, duration and quality, aggravating and alleviating factors, responses to previous treatments, meaning for the patient, and effects on their life.

In the Objective section, the provider's observations are recorded, including vital signs, physical examination, and test results. Acupuncturists record pulses and other palpation findings, tongue and other visual diagnostic findings, and relevant observations of spirit or affect.

In the Assessment section, the patient's problems are listed by priority, weighing medical urgency and the patient's priorities. Each problem is then described, with indications of severity, acuteness or chronicity, risks, causes, and current status of the disease and its progression. Diagnostic impressions are entered, as are potential diagnoses that have been, or need to be, ruled out.

The Plan section contains a record of the treatment performed, and directions for future care and follow-up. Describe all therapeutic interventions, patient and family education, and specify follow-up visit plans. Record medical tests ordered or advised, and the rationale for the tests. If referring the patient, identify to whom, where and when, and supply a reason for the referral.

Authorship of medical record entries must be provided. Every entry should be signed by its author. If transcription is used, the clinician authenticates the entry as accurate by initialing it.

Medical records should be written contemporaneously with the provision of service. They are best written or recorded immediately after treatment, or at least by the end of the same day.

Medical records should be legible, and some states require that they be written in English. Sloppy charting give juries the impression of poor standards of practice. Typewritten charting notes are preferable. Computer speech recognition and transcription software is rapidly improving, and may soon become a reliable means of generating printed chart entries. (See Resources.)

Because medical records are legal records, <u>no entries may be altered or obscured</u>. In legal proceedings, altered medical records are used to suggest an intent to cover up significant facts in the record. In the event of a charting error, circle the error or draw a single thin line through the error in such a way that it can still be read. Write ERROR to the side and then add the date, time and your initials by this entry. Reference where the correction of the error is to be found. Explain the error in detail, and indicate the correction. Only the person who made the error should correct it in the chart.

Risk Control Strategies:
Medical records should be complete, legible, in English, contemporaneously prepared, and signed.

Use the SOAP notes format to record each patient visit.

Never obscure or delete chart entries.

Chart corrections should only be entered by the individual who made the erroneous entry.

Medical Record Confidentiality & Release

Risks:
Breach of duty to maintain medical record confidentiality.

Discussion:
Medical record confidentiality is a right owned by each patient. With certain exceptions, the release of records without waiver of that right by the patient is legally actionable as a breach of privacy.

Let us examine some of those exceptions. If other providers in the same institution have a legitimate need to know the contents of a patient's chart, that information may be shared without patient waiver. These other providers are then bound by the duty of confidentiality. Licensing and accrediting bodies in some states have a right to access medical records to assess charting and care. In a few states, the patient's employer has a right of access to their chart without a waiver, for related workers compensation claims.

There may also be mandatory reporting laws, requiring healthcare providers to report to state agencies in cases involving child or elder abuse, weapons injuries, sexually transmitted diseases (STD's), and other communicable diseases such as tuberculosis. Such reporting mandates do not require patient consent.

Finally, courts may gain access to copies of all or portions of a patient's medical records by court order or *subpoena duces tecum*. In this event, contact an attorney for advice on how to proceed. Even when subpoenaed, portions of the record may be protected.

It is essential to know the access and reporting requirements that apply to acupuncturists in your state, and to update that information at least annually. State acupuncture associations are a natural locus for obtaining and supplying this information on the basis of legal counsel.

Barring previously noted exceptions, a written release form is used to document the patient's waiver of confidentiality for transmission of their records to another party. That release should be filed in the patient's chart, with the date and means of actual transmission.

The standard release form should:

* be addressed to the acupuncturist or practice directed to release information.

* identify the patient.

* define what information is to be released.

Ch.7 Records & Billing

* authorize the release.

* identify who is to receive the information.

* identify a time limit for the authorization (90 days maximum).

* contain the patient's dated signature.

Certain portions of the medical record are accorded an exceptional level of confidentiality. Records associated with drug and alcohol treatment programs; mental health care; and STD's (particularly HIV) require specific release consent by the patient. (42 USC 290 dd-3 & ee-3) Your release form could have boxes to check for the patient to specify the types of information authorized for release. In addition to the contents of the standard release form, substance abuse releases must identify:

* the purpose of the disclosure.

* the nature and extent of information to be disclosed.

* statement that consent may be revoked at any time (although it may have been previously acted upon).

* the date or conditions of expiration of the consent, if not previously revoked.

(42CFR Ch.1, Pt. 2 1992)

Requests for medical records and releases that do not name these most protected informational areas should not have them included. One way to accomplish this is to chart such information in separate sections of the record. Another approach is to cover such information during photocopying. Include a note to the effect that only those portions of the record authorized for release have been included.

Requests for any patient information related to these protected areas must be handled discreetly. A sterling standard practice in substance abuse, mental health and STD clinics is the polite refusal to confirm or deny that a person is a patient, in response to any inquiry.

Most commonly, records are mailed. If they are faxed, it is good practice to include a cover letter which includes directions for the recipient in case the records have arrived at the wrong location. Recipients should be told that confidential records are appended; that the sender should be informed immediately of erroneous receipt; that they should maintain the confidentiality of the records; and that they should return the records by mail or should shred them.

Transmission of records by e-mail is best done in encrypted form. Verbal transmission of patient information by telephone should be preceded by signed patient release, and by verification of the name and position of the recipient. Enter this information in the patient's chart.

Patients have a right of access to the information in their record, but the record itself is the healthcare provider's property. Only copies should be released, and not the original record. By custom, no fee is charged for records sent to other healthcare providers. Attorneys are billed a nominal fee for copies of records.

A final aspect of confidentiality relates to records security. A small acupuncture practice might consider storing records in locking file cabinets. If medical records are computerized, use a password to protect access. Maintain backup copies of computerized records, updated daily and stored securely.

Risk Control Strategies:
Learn and annually update the medical records access and reporting requirements that apply to acupuncturists in your state.

Share patient information with providers and staff only on a need-to-know basis.

Require signed authorization for all (non-mandated) releases of patient records.

Require specific consents for release of records associated with drug & alcohol treatment programs; mental health care; and STD's.

Refuse to confirm or deny that a person is a patient, in response to any inquiries at substance abuse, mental health and STD clinics.

Chart time, date and means of record transmission.

Send copies - never release the original record.

Medical Record Retention & Destruction

Risks:
Breach of duty to maintain medical records for mandated duration.
Breach of confidentiality by improper destruction of records.

Discussion:

States regulate the length of time medical records must be retained. They also define the conditions for the transfer and disposal of medical records.

When a practice is sold to a new owner, the transfer of medical records (and the responsibility for their retention) should be included as an item in the sales agreement. Notify former patients of such a transfer by letter, perhaps augmented by a notice in the local newspaper. Certain states require notification of the acupuncture licensing board when records are transferred.

When medical records are slated for disposal, never dispose of them intact into the garbage or recycling, as confidentiality could be breached. Shred or burn disposed records. Note that the duty of confidentiality does not end, enduring even after the death of a patient! Records of cases actively involved in litigation should not be destroyed. Make a document identifying destroyed charts, along with the notation that they were destroyed in the normal course of business.

Risk Control Strategies:

Retain medical records as required by state regulations.

Document medical record transfers with the sale of a practice.

Shred or burn charts that are to be disposed.

Treatment Limits & Billing Limits

Risks:

Breach of fiduciary duty to patients by over-extending treatment.

Discussion:
How much acupuncture treatment is appropriate? This is a complex matter of professional judgment. One must take into account the medical benefits resulting from acupuncture, potential benefits of other therapies, the costs of acupuncture, the risks involved, and the psychologic effects of continuing or halting treatment. There is no formula for such a calculation. The reasoning that enters into it should be noted in the patient's chart. It is very useful to periodically elicit the patient's perspective of costs and benefits, in mutually developing a plan of treatment.

There is a duty to reasonably limit treatment to what is most beneficial for the patient, and (by extension) to attempt to provide benefits commensurate with costs. When acupuncturists fail to provide significant benefits, they are expected to consider referrals to other providers and to cease acupuncture treatment. Prolonged treatment without progress may be interpreted as self-serving rather than patient-serving.

In the case of third party payers, the treatment limit calculation often becomes simplified. Insurance companies are generally unwilling to pay for treatments that are not 'medically necessary'. Medical necessity is sometimes operatively defined as a maximum number of treatments, or by a cost ceiling for a given diagnostic code. While such arbitrary definitions protect the insurer, they may bear little relationship to the needs of the patient. Providers are torn between their agreements with an insurance company and their desire to serve patients.

The temptation may be to extend covered treatment by billing using another diagnostic code, when the first code has reached a reimbursement limit. Unfortunately, this practice creates another disease or injury of record, another pre-existing condition for the patient, which may later cost them dearly.

Consider this scenario: a patient with a primary complaint of headaches reaches the end of covered treatment, but requires further treatment. Preferring not to pay out of pocket, the patient admits to some very minor back pain. The acupuncturist, wanting to do his best for the patient, agrees to bill continuing treatments under the diagnostic code for back pain as a way of extending reimbursed care for the headaches. Some time later the patient sustains a back injury, perhaps at work or in a motor vehicle accident. Their claim of damages is substantially reduced because of the insurance record of pre-existing back pain.

The ethical high road requires acceptance of insurance reimbursement limits as part of the price of receiving third party reimbursement. Patients may not relish continuing acupuncture as an out of pocket expense, but many will opt to do so if they are experiencing significant benefit.

Risk Control Strategies:
Regularly chart progress (or its lack), and the reasoning that justifies continuation, transfer or cessation of care.

Periodically elicit patient perspectives on costs and benefits of continuing care.

Attempt to provide benefits commensurate with costs, and avoid excessive treatment.

Accept insurance reimbursement limits without resort to marginally warranted diagnostic codes.

Ethical Billing Practices

Risks:
Financial misunderstandings and disagreements.
Liability for unethical or fraudulent billing practices.

Discussion:
Communicate fees for treatment and payment policies to all new patients at the time they arrange for their initial appointment. Address these subjects explicitly in a written information packet supplied to new patients.

Clear communications and well documented accounting records can prevent financial misunderstandings. Maintain patient account records separate from their medical records. Manual and computerized medical accounting systems are readily available. Make backup copies of computerized records at least daily. Keep a daily appointment log and consider having patients sign a daily roster as additional evidence that they arrived for an appointment. These logs are also vital resources in tracing cases in the aftermath of an outbreak of a contagious illness such as HBV.

The acupuncturist is obligated to price her services in some uniform manner, such that no similar purchaser is discriminated against. It is permissible to offer a sliding fee scale to accommodate patients with limited incomes.

Do not bill patients with insurance coverage at a higher rate than other billed patients. Given that insurance reimbursement is frequently slow and paperwork intensive, there is an understandable desire to charge insurers a higher rate. This is not an ethical or legal response. Providers may, however, offer a discount to all patients who pay for services at time of treatment. All who are billed would not receive the discount.

If it is your office policy to charge interest on overdue accounts, the monthly and annual interest rates must be stated in your fee schedule. Maximum interest rates are set by each state.

It is fraudulent to bill third party payers (and particularly those not covering acupuncture services, e.g. Medicare) in ways that intentionally obscure the fact that acupuncture was the primary service provided. Several providers have learned this the hard way.

Risk Control Strategies:
Communicate fees for treatment and payment policies to all new patients at the time they arrange for an initial appointment.

Provide every new patient with a written fee schedule listing all fees and payment policies.

Maintain patient account records separate from medical records.

Account records should be in a standard format, legible and current.

Keep a daily appointment log and signed attendance roster.

Do not bill insurers at a rate higher than for other billed patients.

Do not obscure the fact of acupuncture treatment when billing.

Collection Practices

Risks:
Liability for illegal bill collection practices.

Discussion:
Occasionally patients fail to pay their bills. Of the several recourses available, the most expedient is to write off bad debts as part of the price of doing business, after receiving no response to several bills and to a written request to contact the office to discuss payment. This generosity minimizes the ill will that accompanies collection efforts. A dissatisfied patient who refuses to pay their bill may be spurred by collection efforts to file suit against you for malpractice. Your legal defense will cost far more than any outstanding debt owed to you.

Delinquent accounts can be sent to a reputable collection agency. Advise those accounts in writing that this action will occur, and what conditions are necessary to prevent it. Finally, you may sue in small claims court to receive payment.

At no time and in no way should you (or your collection agency) verbally harass or threaten a debtor. Frequent calls to the debtors home (i.e. more than once a week) is an illegal collection practice in certain states. Calls to the debtor's place of employment, or to their employer, may also be illegal practices. (OMA 1994)

The wisest recourse is to bill delinquent accounts for a period of time, send an overdue account letter, and in the absence of any payment, write off the loss.

Risk Control Strategies:
Bill delinquent accounts for a period of time, send an overdue account letter, and in the absence of payment, write off the loss.

Procedure Codes

Risks:
Liability for unethical or fraudulent billing practices.

Discussion:
Insurance claim forms require entry of standard codes for the medical procedures that are being billed, yet standard codes for acupuncture are not commonplace. Procedure codes are defined in <u>Physicians' Current Procedural Terminology</u> ('CPT 1996') by the American Medical Association. (AMA 1996a) While there are no codes to date for acupuncture, there is indication that the AMA will publish codes for acupuncture and electroacupuncture in 1998. (CSOM 1997a) Until their official appearance, acupuncture is commonly written in next to the 'unlisted physical medicine service or procedure' code, **97799**.

The CPT physical medicine section includes codes for Modalities, Therapeutic Procedures, and Tests & Measurements. Modalities are defined as physical agents (heat, light, sound, electricity) applied for therapeutic reasons. Different modality codes are applied to reflect whether the provider is, or is not, in constant attendance. Procedures are defined as the application of clinical skills or services. These presume constant attendance.

Several acupuncture-related interventions are similar to physical therapy modalities and procedures. Given the lack of acupuncture specific codes, the use of these codes is a good faith attempt to closely represent the actual interventions. For example:

    97010 Hot/Cold Packs (modality, unattended)

    97014 Electrical Stimulation (modality, unattended)

    97026 Infrared (modality, attended)

    97032 Electrical Stimulation (modality, attended)

    97039 Unlisted Modality (modality, attended)

    97124 Massage (procedure)

    97799 Unlisted Physical Medicine Service or Procedure

Transcutaneous electrical nerve stimulation (TENS) is classified under Neurostimulators, Peripheral Nerve, and coded as **64550**. We hesitate to report a code for Vasopneumatic Devices **97016** (modality, attended). Although the term well describes cupping, its common use is probably related to pneumatic stockings that assist venous return in bedridden patients.

There are also CPT codes for new and established patient office visits, varying by the complexity and duration of the visit, but without indication of any procedures. These codes are properly used to bill for evaluation and case management. They should not be used in lieu of acupuncture codes, when acupuncture was the primary purpose of the visit. To do so would obscure the nature of the actual intervention, and could be considered fraudulent billing. If 'office visit' charges are billed to insurers, then they should be billed to all patients similarly. List any such charges in your written fee schedule.

California has developed a set of Workers Compensation codes for acupuncture procedures. (CSOM 1997b) These codes are not applicable to any other billing context. To date they include:

    97800 Acupuncture

    97801 Acupuncture + Electric Stimulation

    97802 Cupping

    97803 Moxibustion

Risk Control Strategies:
CPT codes for acupuncture and electroacupuncture are expected in 1998. Until then, it is common practice to write in 'Acupuncture' next to the unlisted physical medicine service code, 97799.

Do not obscure the fact of acupuncture treatment through evaluation and management (e.g. 'office visit') billing codes.

If 'office visit' charges are billed to insurers, then they should be billed to all patients similarly. List these charges in your written fee schedule.

Diagnostic Codes & Scope Of Practice

Risks:
Exceeding scope of practice by billing with biomedical diagnostic codes and by charting undocumented biomedical diagnoses.

Discussion:

Insurance claim forms require a biomedical diagnostic code from the <u>International Classification of Diseases, 9th Revision, Clinical Modification, 4th Edition</u> ('ICD-9 CM') as a basis for reimbursement. (AMA 1996b) Acupuncturists generally do not have the legal scope of practice to make biomedical diagnoses, and reimbursers are unlikely to accept TOM diagnoses. How can this conflict be resolved?

The language of disease is at once a folk language and several professional languages emanating from various disciplines of care. Certain disease terms are used in both folk and professional contexts. For example, low back pain, neck pain and headache are each simultaneously folk terms and professional terms with diagnostic codes. Lumbar disc degeneration, cervical osteo-arthritis, and migraine headaches are more specialized biomedical diagnostic terms. They are disease diagnoses, whereas folk terms are reports of symptoms and signs. It is beyond the legal scope of most acupuncturists to make biomedical disease diagnoses.

If people are compelled to communicate, then folk language cannot be prohibited. Select diagnostic codes assigned to symptoms and signs, to remain in the province of folk language and to minimize the risk of making unauthorized biomedical diagnoses.

When the acupuncturist has access to the patient's written biomedical diagnosis from a biomedical provider, they may use that diagnosis in diagnostic codes on bills, if it reflects the patient's current condition. It may be used because the acupuncturist is not making the diagnosis, but only reporting a documented diagnosis made by a biomedical provider. Include a copy of the supporting biomedical diagnostic report in the patient's medical record.

Some care in charting is called for in this regard. Couch biomedical diagnoses in presumptive language when lacking a copy of a biomedical report establishing the diagnosis. For example, in the absence of a confirming biomedical report, charting 'Patient presents with a history of right sided headaches which he states have been diagnosed as migraines' provides a more accurate depiction of our knowledge than comes from charting 'Patient presents with a history of right sided migraine headaches'. When unable to document a biomedical diagnosis from a biomedical provider, acupuncturists commit a 'scope error' in asserting such a diagnosis, whether or not they are factually correct.

It is critically important to avoid applying psychologic diagnoses to patients, either in billing or in charting, in the absence of a psychologic or psychiatric referral accompanied by a current diagnosis. Folk language and TOM use of the term 'depression' are not equivalent to the psychologic diagnosis of depression. Entering this diagnosis on an insurance bill gives the patient a record of psychologic disturbance and treatment. This may later be used to deny them employment, insurance, etc. What acupuncturists perceive and respond to as affective depression in the context of TOM might be sub-clinical in the context of psychology. Attention to the patient's affective status is necessary, but one must also use discretion in charting and billing, given the negative social values attached to mental problems. Because the term 'depression' may be misconstrued, it is better to use other terms in charting dejection, gloom or subdued affect. The ancient medical term melancholy serves well. At the opposite end of the spectrum, 'manic' is a psychologic diagnostic term which can be replaced with descriptive but non-diagnostic terms such as dynamic, animated or exhilarated. Refer to Chapter 8 for related discussions of diagnostic and prognostic labeling, and the scope of advice.

With careful phrasing one can indicate diagnostic reasoning, while studiously avoiding personal assertion of biomedical diagnoses. An acupuncturist might note 'The patient's headaches are consistent with a diagnosis of migraine in the following regards:....', without ever stating that the patient has migraine headaches, and without billing using the diagnostic code for migraines.

On the one hand, it is necessary to address the patient's biomedical status and condition, while on the other, acupuncturists are somewhat restricted from doing so by their legal scope of practices. This unavoidable and enduring conflict offers no easy resolution.

Risk Control Strategies:
Select diagnostic codes related to symptoms and signs, unless there is documentation of a current biomedical diagnosis from a biomedical provider.

Avoid the novel assertion of biomedical and psychological diagnoses.

CHAPTER 8

MEDICAL ADVICE

The context of Medical Advice raises issues of the advice given at the initiation of a provider/patient relationship; scope of advice as related to scope of practice; legal hazards of guarantees of outcome; the informed consent process; diagnostic & prognostic labeling; and professional relationships.

Initial Advice

Risks:
Liability for medical advice leading to patient harm.

Discussion:
A patient/practitioner relationship exists if a person directs or changes their health care actions based on a medical provider's advice. (OMA 1994; McWay 1997) A prospective patient's initial telephone inquiry is capable of constituting a patient/practitioner relationship - if medical advice is given - even though the receptionist (and not the practitioner) may have spoken with the caller. Similarly, the medical advice an acupuncturist casually dispenses to an acquaintance at a social event can be interpreted as creating a patient/practitioner relationship...and its potential liabilities. Establishing the existence of such a relationship is necessary to support a legal finding of negligence.

A claim of patient/practitioner relationship based on casual advice may be contestable. But when a person seeks medical services and a provider offers them, the existence of a patient/practitioner relationship is unequivocal, irrespective of whether fees are paid.

To avoid the gratuitous creation of patient/practitioner relationships, the risk control strategy is to *minimize medical advice to that which is prudent and necessary*. To implement this strategy, train your reception staff regarding initial telephone advice.

Telephone triage is required to distinguish between cases appropriate for acupuncture and those not appropriate, as well as to distinguish between medical emergency, urgency, and cases suitable to the routine office visit time frame. Computer software assists telephone triage staff at some institutions. (See Resources)

A knowledge of appropriate referrals is essential. Reception staff should recognize symptoms of heart attacks, and should not overlook the potentially life-threatening nature of asthma attacks. Some guidance comes from listening to the level of concern and stability in the caller's voice. Suggest more than one name for non-emergency medical referrals for callers who are not your patients: you are not making a formal referral of a patient, and do not want the liability associated with a direct professional referral. Providing a caller with options decreases that risk. (Alton 1977)

An outline of a basic telephone protocol follows:

- * Maintain a timed & dated log with a brief summary of each incoming and outgoing telephone call.

- * Respect confidentiality of calls, keeping intra-office discussions on a need-to-know basis.

- * Speak courteously, and listen attentively to the caller's concerns.

Ch.8   Medical Advice   101

* Identify the office and clearly state your own name and position.

* Learn the identity of the caller.

* Learn the purpose of the call.

* Establish the relative urgency of the call.

* Provide appropriate referrals for emergencies and for conditions not suitable for acupuncture treatment. Otherwise, do not give medical advice. Do not provide medical diagnoses.

* Suggest more than one provider for non-emergency medical referrals for non-patients.

* Decide whether (and in what time frame) the acupuncturist should be consulted for advice.

* Determine source of each new patient referral.

* Inform potential new patients of the nature and limits of the practice.

* Inform potential new patients of the fee and payment expectations of the practice.

* Inform potential new patients of the office's appointment cancellation policy. Obtain their home and office telephone numbers (in case the office might unexpectedly need to change the appointment).

* Inform new patients of the location of the office, and of any handicapped access limitations.

* Never make any guarantee of medical outcome.

* Never release patient information over the telephone without specific written authorization from the patient, verification of the recipient's identity, and notation of the call in the patient's chart. The same caveats apply to faxes of patient information, which should be accompanied by a confidentiality notice.

* Take and prioritize messages for the acupuncturist.

The acupuncturist makes tacit decisions to form and continue patient/practitioner relationships. Use discretion to actively select and retain the patients most appropriate to your practice.

Risk Control Strategies:
Train reception staff in telephone triage, and prepare a medical emergency referral list.

Train reception staff in telephone protocol. Instruct which calls to refer directly to you.

Train reception and acupuncture staff to carefully minimize medical advice to that which is prudent and necessary.

Actively select and retain the patients most appropriate to your practice.

Scope Of Advice

Risks:
Advice beyond legal scope; wrong or missed biomedical diagnoses.

Discussion:
It is perilously easy to allow medical advice to overreach legal scope of practice. Patients seek advice about biomedical procedures or medications, and practitioners may hold strong opinions. If you deem it appropriate to share your opinions on biomedical topics, preface, conclude and chart your statements with a suitable disclaimer. For example, you might say 'That matter is outside my training and scope of practice, and so I cannot professionally advise you. I suggest you consult with your biomedical primary care provider. I will offer my personal perspective with you, as long as you understand that it is not given as professional advice.'

Even with such a disclaimer, it is important to recognize limits on the scope and content of advice. *One cannot entirely separate personal advice from the professional context in which it is given.* This is an example of the intrinsic nature of a professional role, and of the accountability that accompanies it. Beyond the issue of scope, erroneous and missed biomedical diagnoses invite liability.

Risk Control Strategies:
Limit medical advice to TOM.

Refer biomedical questions to biomedical practitioners, and refer patients for biomedical diagnosis as prudent.

Guarantees Of Outcome

Risks:
Liability for failure to provide a guaranteed outcome.

Discussion:
Real or implied guarantees of outcome create a contractual obligation to provide them. Should the practitioner offer a guarantee and not provide the outcome, she is liable for a breach of contract. For instance, if an acupuncturist advertises (or states) that she guarantees patients who come for smoking cessation treatments will stop smoking within one week, then she has created a contractual liability if the patient does not succeed in quitting. Such ads may also violate state regulations and scope of practice guidelines related to improper advertising and inducements to care.

Implied guarantees can be much more subtle, but just as risky. Books of glowing testimonials in the waiting room, and/or the use of testimonials in ads, have at times been legally interpreted as implied guarantees of outcome.

It is good practice to share an estimation of the odds of being therapeutically effective, and there is an informed consent duty to do so. However, it is wise to temper that information by sharing the understanding that the practitioner does not know with certainty what the outcome will be for the individual patient before them. One might instill hope when appropriate, and yet honor the ambiguity of each case.

Risk Control Strategies:
Avoid all real and implied guarantees of outcome in ads, waiting room materials, in receptionist's advice to patients, and in your own conversations with patients.

In the information packet supplied to new patients, explicitly disclaim guarantees of outcome: 'As is the case with all types of medical therapies, no guarantees of outcome are made or implied'.

Informed Consent

Risks:
Failure to obtain informed consent for a medical procedure renders the practitioner liable in the event of an adverse outcome, even in the absence of negligence. The practitioner may be liable for battery (unauthorized touch).

Discussion:
Informed consent is an educational process. Practitioners have a legal duty to obtain patient consent prior to treatment. A signed written consent form (express consent) generates strong legal evidence of the consent process, and is required before treatment in many states. However, the form does not constitute the process.

Informed consent ideally supports a patient-centered locus of control over medical choices. The provider educates the patient in medical options so that the patient can select a course of action.

The content and form of the consent process vary from state to state. Basic elements of informed consent are given by **Table 8.1.**

The acupuncturist must explain to the patient the nature of proposed *Procedures*. For example, she would describe needling, including the approximate number of needles to be used, the duration of needle insertion, needle manipulation, and the sensations and level of discomfort involved. She should identify the patient's TOM diagnosis, and include her sense of the benefits

ELEMENTS OF INFORMED CONSENT

> 1. Procedure
>
> 2. Alternatives
>
> 3. Risks
>
> 4. Query need for more information

Table 8.1

and prospects for a successful outcome, and the <u>prognosis for the patient if the procedure is not performed</u>.

The acupuncturist must present treatment *Alternatives* - such other therapeutic options as may be available to the patient. In the case of a back sprain, she could state 'You might consider physical therapy or chiropractic as other ways to treat your back pain'.

The acupuncturist must describe the *Risks* of the procedure. Concerning potentially serious injuries, she must advise patients of all but the most remote. Concerning potentially slight injuries, she must advise patients of those most likely to occur. If a reasonable person in circumstances similar to the patient's would consider a risk significant, then that risk should be presented. A thorough disclosure of risks reduces practitioner liability.

Finally, she must *Query* whether the patient desires any further information, and offer a more detailed discussion as requested. Not all states require the query, but it is good practice.

When should one use a written consent form signed by the patient? This <u>must</u> be done for all research with human subjects. It is also required for procedures that alter the physical structure of the body, such as surgery. A very conservative reading might include direct moxibustion is this category, as it leaves a scar. For a definitive position, consult your state statutes, licensing board, and professional association.

Use written consent for interventions which use devices not cleared for marketing by the FDA. This may include electroacupuncture, direct and indirect moxibustion, cupping, coining, acupressure, lasers and magnets. (Refer to Chapter 12.)

The most cautious legal perspective suggests that express consent be used routinely for all medical interventions, as the consent document is often the only credible evidence that a patient has been advised of the risks of treatment and has given their consent. Such a formal approach may generate patient anxiety, where other local medical practitioners do not routinely use written consent.

Whether using a written form in addition to the consent conversation or not, document and date the informed consent conference in the patient's chart. This may be done with the brief notation **PAR**, which can be underlined **<u>PAR</u>** to denote a more detailed discussion occurred in response to a Query about the need for more information. (OMA 1994) Or you may choose to chart a fuller description of the consent conversation, which is preferable from a legal standpoint.

Risk Control Strategies:
Supply new patients with written materials which accurately describe each type of therapeutic intervention you do. These materials should also thoroughly disclose risks of treatment.

Discuss each procedure that is new to a patient, using the P-A-R-Q protocol.

Chart the informed consent process.

Always use signed written consent for investigational studies.

Use written consent for interventions that use devices not cleared for marketing by the FDA.

Diagnostic & Prognostic Labeling

Risks:
Creation of perceived illness through injudicious diagnostic and prognostic labeling.

Discussion:
Diagnostic and prognostic labeling can lead patients to an unhealthy perception of their condition. This adds to the burden of existing disease processes, or creates anxieties in the absence of disease. Pathogenic labeling is not only a problem of biomedical providers. TOM practitioners are trained in a set of syndrome and imbalance categories, and are quite capable of inflicting 'labeling harm' upon patients, if not conscious of this risk.

Yet labeling can also be reassuring. Patients universally request a name for their condition. (Kleinman 1980) The existence of a name objectifies and reifies the experience of illness, and justifies the sick role. The patient's symptom story is corroborated by a professional diagnosis. Diagnostic labels can contribute to a sense of control for provider and patient - the condition is experienced as less unknown by virtue of having a name.

The art lies in gauging for each patient which labels will help and which labels will harm. Some of what is said to patients seems to pass by unheard; yet other words pierce to the heart, and are carried for years. Have you imparted a message of imbalance in the context of the patient's innate wholeness, or one of pervasive illness in the context of TOM?

For a discussion of charted diagnostic labels, scope of practice, and the negative social value of psychologic diagnoses, see Chapter 7.

Risk Control Strategies:
Apply diagnostic and prognostic labels judiciously, with keen appreciation for the positive and negative potentials of labeling.

Professional Relationships

Risks:
Harming the relationship between a patient and another of their providers; creating ill will among fellow acupuncturists or among other medical professionals; slander; defamation.

Discussion:
The advice given patients regarding the medical care they have received elsewhere requires a very thoughtful selection of words,

particularly when critical of that care. Providers have a protective duty to patients in voicing their concerns in those rare instances when they believe another provider has frankly maltreated the patient. But it is prudent to let the routine professional evaluation of other providers remain for the most part a silent one. A patient may have great trust in the provider you criticize. Voicing negative opinions could harm their relationship, or could lead the patient (and the other provider) to speak poorly of you. At worst, defamatory speech, if untrue, is legally actionable as slander. At best, demeaning other providers creates enduring professional ill will. Guide patients toward preferable sources of medical services for positive reasons, rather than guiding patients away from less appropriate providers for negative reasons.

It is not uncommon to differ with other providers in terms of diagnosis or therapy. Generously affirm the diversity of opinions. If either party is unswayed, then tactfully 'agree to disagree' while remaining professionally respectful.

Risk Control Strategies:
Other than in blatant cases of maltreatment, speak no ill of other providers.

Guide patients toward preferable sources of medical services for positive reasons, rather than guiding patients away from less appropriate providers for negative reasons.

CHAPTER 9

MEDICAL EMERGENCIES

In the context of Medical Emergencies we define common medical emergencies and discusses the need for response protocols and first aid supplies. The chapter closes with discussion of the limits and imperatives of first aid response.

Common Medical Emergencies

Risks:
Patient harm from failure to recognize or respond appropriately to medical emergencies.

Discussion:
Medical emergencies happen unexpectedly, and could occur in your office. They may - or may not - be related to the medical procedures the patient is undergoing. Preparation for response begins with training. Several states require the acupuncturist to maintain current CPR training. It is beyond the scope of this text to teach first aid. The reader is advised to consult texts dedicated to that topic. (Bergeron 1987; Malamed 1987)

All employees designated as first aid responders have bloodborne pathogen exposure risks. Employers must fulfill every requirement of the OSHA Bloodborne Pathogen Standard for designated first aid responders. Refer to Chapter 6.

Though unexpected, medical emergencies are not entirely unpredictable. ***Table 9.1*** lists common medical emergencies.

MEDICAL EMERGENCIES

Heart Attack Stroke	
Seizures	**Diabetic Reactions**
Pneumothorax	**Bleeding**
Asthma Attack	**Choking**
Vomiting	**Abdominal Pain**
Fainting	**Broken Needle**
Anaphylaxis & Allergic Reactions	

Table 9.1

Develop a written response protocol for each of the above problems. In those protocols, identify the necessary equipment and supplies. Then obtain and organize all medical emergency response equipment. Clearly indicate locations of first aid equipment, and inform employees. Regularly inventory and replenish the first aid kit, and inspect for blood or OPIM contamination.

Two PPE items are essential for the acupuncture first aid kit. The first item is latex gloves. Whenever there is bleeding, first aid responders must put on gloves before attending to the person in need. In this situation, first aid responders should prevent others from intervening until they also don gloves.

The second PPE item is some type of resuscitation barrier - either a disposable mouth shield or a ventilation bag. The former shields the provider from direct contact with mouth fluids during mouth-to-mouth breathing, while the latter circumvents mouth contact altogether by means of a patient face mask connected to a hand operated air bag.

Beyond PPE and basic first aid supplies, include a sturdy splinter forceps, used to grip and remove a protruding needle shaft fragment in the very rare event of needle breakage. Also include a one page summary of CPR techniques as a memory refresher.

Among emergencies directly related to acupuncture, fainting is probably the most common and most preventable. Fainting is not necessarily an innocuous event. Serious head injuries and permanent damages have been caused by fainting during minor medical procedures. Patient positioning is the primary key to prevention. If patients are reclined, supine or prone for treatment, they are less likely to faint, and should they faint, they are less likely to fall. Leaving patients unattended with needles inserted, and with the patients seated on a table or chair, is an invitation to grievous fainting incidents.

When needling a seated patient, be in constant attendance, elicit verbal feedback on how the patient is feeling, and maintain visual assessment of the patient's facial color. Sudden paleness, thirst, nausea, dizziness, and/or visual disturbances often precede fainting. Be alert to these symptoms, rapidly remove needles, and safely recline the patient.

Risk Control Strategies:
Prepare a response protocol for common medical emergencies.

Periodically update and review emergency response protocols.

Obtain and organize medical emergency response supplies; highlight location with a sign.

Regularly inventory and replenish the first aid kit and inspect for blood or OPIM contamination.

Maintain current CPR training.

Position patients in a reclined, supine or prone position for acupuncture whenever practical.

When needling a seated patient, be in constant attendance, elicit verbal feedback, and maintain visual assessment.

Limits Of First Aid Response

Risks:
Liability for practicing beyond training and competency.

Discussion:
Interveners in medical emergencies are to some extent shielded from liability by Good Samaritan laws. But Good Samaritan laws

primarily apply to emergencies outside the clinical workplace. Providers are liable for reckless, incompetent, or sub-standard emergency medical responses in the clinic. Equipment and techniques used in emergency response are expected to be used correctly. Providers must use discretion in defining the limits of response. Fortunately, in most settings emergency medical services can be summoned by dialing **911** or a local emergency number. Making that call is the first item in response protocols for serious emergencies, followed by the interim provision of supportive care.

Providers are morally compelled to intervene to protect life in the interim, in cases such as cardiac arrest, airway obstruction or copious bleeding. When doing CPR, it is possible to fracture ribs. This is an acknowledged risk of the procedure, and such an outcome is difficult to conclusively attribute to malpractice. If trained in CPR, then the imperative to protect life by doing CPR when necessary easily outweighs other liability concerns.

Risk Control Strategies:
Use discretion in defining the limits of personal emergency response.

Telephone for help (**911** or local emergency number) as the first step in response to serious medical emergencies.

Next to every clinic telephone, post the phone numbers for the nearest hospital emergency room, and for the post-exposure medical provider.

CHAPTER 10

INTERPERSONAL ASPECTS OF TREATMENT

The context of Interpersonal Aspects of Treatment brings us to issues of the therapeutic relationship; rapport; privacy & modesty; and sexual boundaries.

The Therapeutic Relationship

Risks:
Inability to develop the healing potential of a therapeutic relationship; re-definition of the therapeutic relationship by transference and counter-transference.

Discussion:
The relationship between provider and patient is neither simple, static nor singular. Consider these three components of a therapeutic relationship - the *role relationship*, the *real relationship*, and the *projected relationship*.

The role relationship encompasses much of what is done within the context of a social contract. People with problems adopt various sick and patient roles, and providers enact socially defined caregiver roles. In the patient role, people arrange and pay for appointments, share their woes, and submit to some extent to the diagnostics and therapeutics of providers. Provider role duties include compassionate behavior, professional knowledge and technical skill in the provision of care. Certain role duties are codified by law (e.g. confidentiality; sexual boundaries).

The core of the social contract contains the real essence of why parties engage in the role relationship. Patients intend to gain an aspect of healing at some cost. Providers intend to convey an aspect of healing at some gain. This intended exchange frames the boundaries of the real relationship.

Within those boundaries, and infusing the role actions, are the energetic presences of patient and provider. The <u>real relationship</u> consists of the qualities of being manifested in the meeting of patient and provider. The real relationship is an interchange of Jing-Shen (essence-spirit), conducted within the limiting circumstances of the core social contract.

The real relationship is modified by the <u>projected relationship</u>, which consists of transferences, counter-transferences and implicit expectations involving patient and provider. In transference, the patient 'mistakes' the provider as a player in her life, beyond the confines of the social contract of healing. The provider may be projected as a father or mother figure, a brother or sister, a lover or a combatant. In counter-transference, the provider similarly 'mistakes' the patient as a player in his life.

Besides transferences, projections include implicit expectations that alter the boundaries of the social contract. While projections generate useful material in the context of psychoanalysis, they frequently lead medical work astray by subtle unilateral re-definitions of the nature of the relationship.

The <u>therapeutic relationship</u> consists of the continual interplay of role, real, and projected relationships. Artful and authentic providers develop a transcendent healing potential from the role and real relationships. (Novack 1987; Meissner 1992) The patient may experience a deep trust in the provider that even supersedes their faith in the treatment. The provider co-creates that field of trust through a profound (albeit temporary) non-judgmental empathy with and acceptance of the patient's being. This action is both <u>role</u> and <u>real</u>. Taking it as primarily real (and not role-delimited) sustains transference and counter-transference.

Witnessing the dynamics of the therapeutic relationship facilitates the ability to direct and develop it's healing potentials, while avoiding the interpersonal entanglements of projection.

Risk Control Strategies:
Recognize the dynamics of the therapeutic relationship to direct and develop its healing potentials and to avoid interpersonal entanglements.

Rapport

Risks:
Lack of rapport increases dissatisfaction and malpractice actions.

Discussion:
The therapeutic relationship is an extension of rapport between patient and provider. (Rosenzweig 1993) One of the best ways to build that rapport is by taking the time to listen to patients' illness narratives. It is innately healing to be well heard, to tell the story of one's illness just as it has been experienced, and to share this narrative with an empathetic listener. Patients require (and easily recognize) a safe environment where they do not feel compelled to censor, deform or compress their story. It is a signal honor to be granted access to genuine stories, and to share some in return.

Physicians have recently become more aware of the importance of rapport. Rapport is being addressed in terms of communications skills, such as learning to read and respond to the non-verbal signs of patients' body language. The providers' energetic presence, their participation in an authentic act of <u>real</u> relationship, might well be more fundamental to rapport.

Risk Control Strategies:
Schedule sufficient time to hear patients' authentic illness stories.

Create an environment conducive to developing rapport.

Privacy & Modesty

Risks:
Offense to patients' sensibilities through lack of sensitivity to modesty values.

Discussion:
Expectations of privacy and modesty differ by culture, and differ within a culture by individuals. Robing and disrobing are considered more or less private acts in our culture, and are to be strictly respected as private acts in clinical settings. When patients need to undress to allow access to acupuncture points or areas, give them clear instructions about what clothes may remain on, and provide them with a gown and/or draping sheets. Always knock before entering a treatment area and inquire if the patient is ready, so that you do not intrude on disrobing or robing.

Being naked or exposed in the view of another is similarly an uncomfortable breach of modesty values, particularly when the viewer is of the opposite sex. Yet many medical interventions require some degree of nakedness. Always attempt to minimize viewed nakedness. When asking a mostly naked patient to reposition themselves on the table during treatment, turn away so as not to view them until they have again draped themselves. Whether or not an individual patient expresses discomfort at bodily exposure, always act to protect modesty.

Risk Control Strategies:
Leave the treatment area when patients are to robe or disrobe, so that these actions may be accomplished in privacy. Knock and inquire before entering the room.

Provide gowns, draping sheets, and clear instructions to patients.

Always act to minimize viewed nakedness.

Sexual Boundaries

Risks:
Unethical conduct; perceived sexual impropriety in the absence of impropriety.

Discussion:
Sexual behavior between practitioner and patients is a violation of the practitioner's legal duty to maintain a fiduciary relationship, and it is considered unethical conduct. Medical practitioners are frequently viewed by patients as having greater authority, knowledge and power. A healer may be idealized by patients. Imbalances of power and the extension of regard and trust contribute to patient vulnerability to practitioner sexual advances.

The patient-provider relationship is a fiduciary relationship, which is to say it is one of trust. The practitioner is trusted to act principally in the best interests of the patient, and to take no advantage of patient vulnerability in any way. Regardless of whether sexual behavior is initiated by patient or provider, the provider is always strictly accountable for engaging in sexual behavior with patients. (OR BME 1997)

Occasionally there are seductive patients. The acupuncturist is obliged to redirect the focus of the interaction to their legitimate medical work, with as much tact as possible. Verbally acknowledge seductive behavior, tactfully mention why it is inappropriate, and be willing to discuss the matter. If this is insufficient, set behavioral boundaries (e.g. 'I can't do my work with such a strong sexual dynamic present. I need to have a third party present as we work, or I need to refer you to another provider, if you continue to sexualize our interaction.') If necessary, follow through by using a chaperone or by referring the patient out. Chart thoroughly.

There are instances when sexual impropriety is impugned, even though no impropriety has occurred. Consider the scenario of a male acupuncturist needling Ren 1 on a rebellious female teenager in the privacy of a closed treatment room, with no one else present. Assume that his actions are purely professional, that he explains the procedure before needling, obtains tacit consent, and explains again while needling. Yet afterwards, patient and provider stories of what took place are remarkably different. The acupuncturist could find himself accused of sexual impropriety, with only his word to establish his innocence.

This scenario highlights four contributors to the potential perception of sexual impropriety. The first involves the identity of the patient, who might be extremely vulnerable, frightened by her bodily sensations, rebellious, or wanting the attention and power that results from creating a scene. The second concerns the gender difference of patient and provider. The third contributor is the lack

Ch.10 Interpersonal Aspects Of Treatment

of witnesses. The fourth relates to the choice of points or techniques used.

The strategy of having a chaperone present in the treatment area addresses the first three of the above factors. Consider an alternate selection of points in place of points near the sexual organs as another risk reduction strategy.

Whenever you work on the lower pelvic area of a patient (regardless of gender), put on latex exam gloves first. In addition to the hygienic benefits, the glove barrier psychologically reinforces the perception of the activity as clinical, for both patient and provider.

Risk Control Strategies:
Be aware and in control of your own sexual intent and behavior - refrain from provocative conversation and/or sexual touch, and do not become romantically involved with patients.

Tactfully confront seductive patients.

Have a chaperone present during treatment of patients who you consider at high risk for 'perceived sexual impropriety'.

Inform patients that they may bring a friend with them into the treatment area.

Consider alternate points in place of points near the sexual organs.

Whenever you work on the lower pelvic area of a patient (regardless of gender), put on latex exam gloves first.

CHAPTER 11

LEGAL ASPECTS OF TREATMENT

In the context of Legal Aspects of Treatment we address scope of practice; professional duties & liabilities; negligence; primary care provider status; and the dilemma of non-standard medicine & medical standards of care.

Scope Of Practice

Risks:
Liability for practicing outside legal scope or beyond competency.

Discussion:
Each state regulating acupuncture does so under its own laws defining the scope of practice - <u>what may be done</u> by acupuncturists. The statutes are given operational definition through regulations enacted by state agencies such as licensing boards.

In some jurisdictions, acupuncture associations may have at least quasi-legal authority to regulate portions of their scope of practice, and to define performance standards. Courts have at times considered quasi-legal factors in determining issues of scope. However, engaging in practices beyond those defined in law and regulation entails serious risks.

The definition of what may be done demarcates <u>what may not be done</u>, the regulated limits of diagnostic and therapeutic interventions. To engage in actions beyond one's scope is tacitly illegal and invites regulatory agency reactions, irrespective of any resultant patient harm. For instance, acupuncturists cannot advise patients with regards to prescription medications, because that is beyond their legal scope of practice. It also constitutes practicing medicine without a license.

Do not give the appearance of practicing beyond legal scope. If your scope does not extend to the use of vitamins, homeopathics, minerals, amino acids, etc., then those supplements should neither be displayed nor presented for sale in your office. Their presence invites the risk of prosecution.

Even though scope of practice provisions define what may be done by a licensed acupuncturist, in the absence of competency in all aspects of that scope we discern compelling instances of _what should not be done_. For example, if the legal scope of practice includes the interpretation of biomedical laboratory tests, and yet an individual acupuncturist has no training in that area, then that individual should refrain from interpreting lab tests. Engaging in medical interventions without competency is legally negligent. Competency is demonstrated in practice, and is generated and supported by documentable training. _What may be done_ is not equivalent to _what should be done_, in light of both professional discretion and malpractice case law. Refer to the discussions of Negligence and Primary Care Provider Status below.

Risk Control Strategies:
Obtain, read and file copies of the laws and regulations governing acupuncture in your state. Update annually.

Do not sell products that are outside your scope of practice.

Restrict medical advice and interventions to matters within your scope _and_ competency as supported by training.

Professional Duties & Liabilities

Risks:
Liability for failure to uphold professional duties.

Discussion:
Acupuncture laws and regulations explicitly define some of the professional duties - <u>what must be done</u> by acupuncturists. These include matters such as how acupuncturists identify themselves; license renewal requirements; conditions under which patients must be referred to physicians; and the maintenance of records.

The subject of how acupuncturists identify themselves deserves comment. State requirements vary considerably. Some require that acupuncturists wear a name tag bearing the title 'Licensed Acupuncturist'. States define what letters may, must, or may not be placed after one's name (L.Ac., O.M.D., etc.). It is important to closely follow state law in the use of professional titles and initials. If one presents degrees or titles from another country, that fact must be made clear. For example: 'M.D. (China)' clarifies that the individual is not an M.D. in the U.S.A. Acupuncturists are also advised to practice using the same name that they are licensed under. (OR.BME 1997)

Identification is also at issue when answering the clinic telephone. If you do not possess a doctorate degree, it is more accurate to answer the telephone saying 'Acupuncture, (Jane Doe)'s office', or words to that effect, rather than saying 'Doctor (Doe)'s office'. Portray yourself accurately, and as required by state law.

Beyond specific acupuncture laws, there are legally imposed duties that broadly apply to healthcare providers. Where the law recognizes a duty, it also establishes a liability for failure to perform the duty. A range of professional duties are revealed in three branches of liability law: contract law, intentional torts, and non-intentional torts. (McWay 1997)

Contract law recognizes breach of contract as a liability arising from guarantees of cure that have not been produced, as well as from non-performance in contracts to treat. Oral or written guarantees of cure generate a contractual duty. For this reason providers are careful to avoid explicit or implicit guarantees.

Torts are legal wrongs, usually not criminal actions, for which an injured party may bring suit. Intentional torts are considered to be willful wrongs. They include defamation; invasion of privacy; fraud; abandonment; and assault and battery.

Defamation of character is the harming of a person's reputation. It reflects the duty to avoid harmful words with respect to another's character and skills. The duty is enacted through tactful communication. (See Ch.8, Professional Relationships.)

Invasion of privacy, the dissemination of private or protected information, reflects the duty of confidentiality. (See Ch.7.) Confidentiality is modified by reporting requirements, which reflect the legal duty to release certain information to the state. In California, acupuncturist reporting requirements are identical to those for physicians. Each state has its own requirements.

Fraud involves the intentional deception of another for personal gain. Fraud reflects the duty of honesty. (See Ch.7 and Ch.12.)

Abandonment, the provider's precipitous and unilateral termination of a patient/provider relationship, reflects the duty to provide continuity in care. Normally the relationship is terminated by mutual consent, by lack of need for more treatment, or by the patient's dismissal of the provider. It may also be terminated by the provider with reasonable notice (e.g. 30 days, certified letter) as long as the provider continues to be available during this transition time. A patient may be required to pay for services at time of treatment as a condition of further treatment, but should be informed well in advance if this is a new requirement.

If unilaterally terminating the care of a patient, one does not need to state why, but must indicate the fact of withdrawing from the patient's further professional care as of a given date. If retiring or selling a practice, give written advance notification to patients, to prevent damages related to abandonment. Also provide information on the disposition and availability of patient medical records.

Continuity of care is enhanced by an office policy of making follow-up phone calls to no-show patients to facilitate re-scheduling or to clarify a patient-initiated closure of the relationship. This policy is of particular importance with respect to seriously ill patients.

If you will be unavailable for a period of time (e.g. on vacation), designate a substitute provider, and offer that provider's name and telephone number to all patients who call in your absence.

Assault is threatening to harm, while battery is physical contact without permission or exceeding consent. They are criminal and civil torts. Battery reflects the duty to obtain consent. (See Ch.8).

Non-intentional torts are unintended wrongs, of which the most notable is negligence, considered below. Vicarious liability and failure to warn are other non-intentional torts.

Vicarious liability, the responsibility for actions of a person in our employ, reflects a duty to carefully select, train and direct employees. (See Ch.5.)

Failure to warn reflects the duty to inform persons at risk of harm (and to inform police) if a patient presents a serious threat.

Risk Control Strategies:
Encourage state acupuncture associations to compile and annually update (with help of legal counsel) a list of regulations pertaining to acupuncturists, and to disseminate a concise summary of duties.

Accurately present your name, degrees, titles and acupuncture licenses as directed by state law.

Provide continuity of care with missed appointment calls, substitute provider availability during absences, and advance notification of any withdrawal from provider/patient relationships.

Negligence

Risks:
Liability for negligence in the performance of duties.

Discussion:
Negligence is the liability most commonly cited in support of a claim of malpractice. Negligence broadly reflects the duty of care: to provide a quality of care not below the standard practices of ones peers. Negligence is the failure to act as a reasonably prudent practitioner. It may be substantiated by demonstrating departures from approved practices, and by violations of scope of practice. (Sloan 1992)

COMPONENTS OF NEGLIGENCE

---

1. Patient / Provider Relationship

2. Breach Of Duty

3. Proximate Cause

4. Damages

Table 11.1

Negligence is more narrowly defined as the failure to possess or exercise adequate knowledge, skill, care and/or diligence. The four components needed to support a finding of negligence are presented in **Table 11.1**.

One must first establish that a patient/practitioner relationship existed, and hence that duties of care were present. Then the inquiry would identify the breach of duty. The breach must next be implicated as the proximate cause of damages. Breach of duty may refer to:

* failure to proceed with sufficient education, or failure to keep knowledge current.

* failure to exercise technical skill.

* failure to proceed with reasonable caution and regard for safety.

* failure to be observant and careful.

* failure to proceed in the best interests of the patient.

* failure to obtain informed consent.

* failure to timely refer a patient for other medical consultation.

* engaging in practices beyond legal scope.

A breach of duty may occur due to an omission - something one did not do but should have done, or it may occur due to a commission - something one did incorrectly.

Malpractice, a more encompassing term than negligence, refers to professional misconduct, or not following acceptable standards of care as established by expert testimony. (McWay 1997) Gross negligence means acting with wanton disregard for safety.

Risk Control Strategies:
Uphold adequate standards of practice. Refer to 'Best Practice' recommendations for guidance.

Maintain good patient/practitioner relationships.

Limit practice to what is within your legal scope <u>and</u> competency as supported by demonstrable training.

Err on the side of caution.

Present inherent risks of acupuncture procedures in the informed consent process and in informed consent documents. Note that process in the patient's chart.

Chart patient care thoroughly, legibly and timely. Never obscure or alter a patient medical record.

Obtain professional liability insurance.

Crisis Response Strategies:

First attend to patient emergencies immediately, and always do your best to protect the patient's health. Thereafter contact your professional liability insurance company and attorney, should a serious adverse event have occurred. If you receive a summons and malpractice complaint, or a letter requesting damages be paid, contact your liability insurance company and attorney prior to responding. Do not release original medical records.

Write a narrative account of the event, addressed to your attorney. This protects it as a confidential client-attorney communication. Do not file a copy in with the patient's medical record, but instead file it separately. Provide a detailed summary of the patient's care starting with their initial visit. Explain the rationale of your interventions. If a procedure resulted in injury, describe the procedure and the injury in detail. If medical devices were used, identify their make and model. Identify the roles of other personnel and medical providers involved in caring for the patient, and the nature and tenor of your professional interactions. Describe your own professional training, specialization, practice setting, and length of time in practice. Finally, identify the potential strong and weak points of the case, particularly addressing how your work may have been above or below the standards of acupuncture care.

You may be summoned to a formal deposition meant to discover the facts of the case. You will be questioned under oath, and should answer truthfully, answer without hostility, and most pointedly, <u>carefully answer only the question that was asked and no more</u>.

Be particularly alert for some version of this question from the plaintiff's attorney: *'This outcome does not ordinarily occur if the acupuncturist uses reasonable care, is that correct?'* If you answer in the affirmative, you will have provided expert testimony of your own negligence. A preferable response is: 'The outcome does not ordinarily occur. It's occurrence is primarily related to the inherent risks of the procedure.' However, this can only be stated if truthful. (OMA 1994) The legal process is an intricate one. Obtain legal counsel immediately in the event of a suit or potential suit.

Primary Care Provider Status

Risks:
Liability for incompetent biomedical judgment leading to harm.

Discussion:
Primary care providers (PCP's) are patients' first recourse for professional medical help. PCP's act as 'portals of entry' into the health care system. The PCP commonly assesses the patient, supplies generalist treatment, provides referrals and conducts follow-ups. Most PCP's are biomedically trained and have prescriptive authority. Examples include family practice M.D.'s and osteopathic physicians (D.O.'s). PCP status has only recently been extended to some mid-level providers such as nurse practitioners (N.P.'s). PCP's handle the chores of general medicine, such as the diagnosis and management of asthma, high blood pressure, diabetes, rashes, etc.

PCP status commonly generates a high level of accountability to biomedical standards of diagnosis, treatment and referral. Performance criteria and standard of care expectations for N.P.'s are fundamentally no different than for M.D.'s. Medical specialists are typically not PCP's. Those physician specialists who become designated as PCP's in health maintenance organizations (HMO's) often acquire extensive continuing education to be able to competently perform PCP tasks.

Medical professionals legally defined as PCP's become eligible for third party reimbursement under state or federal law and/or insurance company policy. In HMO's, PCP's frequently receive capitation payments. With the decline of fee for service, third party reimbursement eligibility assumes crucial importance. Reimbursement profoundly shapes professional destiny.

Several states have defined chiropractors (D.C.'s), and naturopaths (N.D.'s) as PCP's. California (in 1978) and New Mexico (in 1997) have designated acupuncturists as PCP's. Because these several professions are not licensed for the full scope of biomedical therapeutics, they cannot be legally authorized or expected to perform standard biomedical interventions. Still at issue are standards of diagnosis and referral.

PCP status provides California acupuncturists with entry into the Workers Compensation insurance system. But PCP acupuncturists may be held to standards for patient examination, diagnosis, referral, charting, assessment and report writing defined not just by other acupuncturists, but by biomedical PCP's and insurers.

California acupuncturists have within their scope of practice the authority to order and interpret biomedical laboratory tests (although they themselves cannot perform phlebotomy, the actual drawing of blood samples). With this scope comes accountability to recognize the need for such tests, to correctly interpret their meaning, and to make timely referrals to biomedical practitioners. One California acupuncturist has already been sued for wrongful death, for having failed to diagnose a cancer which progressed and caused the patient's death eighteen months later.

The nature of primary care expectations will be determined in the courts over many years. Will PCP acupuncturists be held to the same diagnostic and referral standards as biomedical PCP's? Or will they define a more limited 'portal of entry' practice, accountable primarily for appropriate referral?

The impact of PCP status will be determined in some measure by acupuncture colleges, which must supply an advanced level of biomedical diagnostic training to support proficient performance of the requisite kinds of medical judgment. How thoroughly, uniformly, and rapidly will the colleges rise to the occasion?

The public will significantly define PCP acupuncture in the ways they use and understand acupuncture in relation to other available medical services. What types of problems do people choose to bring to PCP acupuncturists as a first recourse for professional care? How satisfied are first recourse acupuncture patients in comparison with first recourse patients from other types of primary care providers? What are the comparative levels of trust in diagnosis and advice? The outcome of these issues largely demarcates acupuncturists' realized liability risks.

The question of competency in an expanded scope of practice is certainly a key one for those acupuncturists who have been 'grandfathered' in to the O.M.D. designation. Despite legal authority to engage in a broader scope of practice, it is negligent to perform actions within that scope without competency, which is usually based on demonstrable training. Self-regulation is a societal expectation placed on professional behavior. Obtaining and documenting additional training is the route to legitimately expand one's actual scope of practice, within an expanded scope granted by law. Continuing education, legislation and litigation over the next several decades will influence the level of competency and the necessity for self-limitation.

PCP status based on biomedical disease diagnosis expectations is but one approach to advanced practice and integration in the health care system. As an alternative, the profession might develop a 'PCP preventive medicine-acupuncturist' with moderate biomedical disease diagnostic skills, but high early intervention and wellness maintenance skills. This model fits the spirit of TOM and the natures of people who become acupuncturists. Recall that health does not primarily emanate from healthcare!

Risk Control Strategies:
PCP acupuncturists: Learn and follow the reporting duties and case law of PCP's in your state.

PCP acupuncturists: Prepare with a strong background in biomedical patient examination, diagnostic testing, differential diagnosis, charting, assessment and report writing.

PCP acupuncturists: Establish close referral relationships with biomedical PCP's, and refer when in doubt about the patient's current biomedical diagnosis.

PCP acupuncturists: Specify on informed consent documents that you are not taking primary responsibility for the patient's biomedical diagnosis.

Do not practice beyond competency and demonstrable training.

Carry professional liability insurance.

Non-Standard Medicine & Standards Of Care

Risks:
Failure to meet implicit and explicit standards of medical care.

Discussion:
The context of laws and regulations rests upon a broader frame of reference - the implicit social standards of medical prudence and responsibility. The acupuncturist must intuit the perspectives of a judge, a review board, or a jury of local residents who might consider their actions in the context of common values and beliefs. Good intentions alone will not suffice as protection in courts of law. One of the most difficult and necessary attainments involves the development of a <u>balanced medical judgment</u> based upon:

- * legal and regulatory contexts.

- * considerations of community standards of care.

- * diagnostic & therapeutic potentials of biomedicine.

- * professional practice standards of biomedicine.

- * diagnostic and therapeutic potentials of TOM.

- * professional practice standards of TOM.

- * the particular needs of the patient before us.

The problem of practicing within community medical standards of care is a complex one, as acupuncture is an inherently foreign perspective, an 'other' standard of practice. In fact, much of the clinical utility of acupuncture derives from its 'otherness'. This constitutes the dilemma of non-standard medicine: providers must deliver other practices in the context of common standards. Tracing the middle way of this delicate passage requires differentiation between greater and lesser medico-legal risks. Medico-legal risks are generated as much by cultural and professional belief systems as they are by biomedicine and law.

The middle way cannot be attained in isolation. Peer review processes help acupuncturists achieve common standards. Acupuncture associations, in dialogue with regulatory agencies, contribute to definitions of professional standards of care and scope of practice. Sharing perspectives beyond the profession's boundaries develops mutual understandings in social, medical and regulatory communities.

Risk Control Strategies:
Develop a sense of medico-legal norms by reading malpractice case law.

Take an active part in the work of your professional associations.

Network with other medical professions.

Chapter 12

FDA Regulations

The context of FDA Regulations open with a review of FDA device standards. This information is then applied to acupuncture devices. The chapter closes with an evaluation of dietary supplement regulations.

FDA Device Standards: Background

Risks:
FDA regulatory compliance; health fraud & malpractice liabilities.

Discussion:
These interpretations of FDA policy comprise an informed reading of regulatory praxis. To keep abreast of device policy, monitor the FDA Center for Devices & Radiological Health (CDRH) Internet website at: **http://www.fda.gov/cdrh**

The FDA regulates promotion and sale of medical devices, while states regulate the practice of medicine. The distinction is not a neat one, as the FDA deems that clinical use of a medical device constitutes sale. Furthermore, FDA rulings are used by other agencies in the determination of reimbursement policies and in the definition of standards of care. FDA policies strongly influence the practice of medicine.

The FDA categorizes 'pre-amendment' medical devices into three classes according to the degree of control required for safety. (Pre-amendment devices are those devices marketed in the USA before the 1976 Amendments to the Food & Drug Act.) Class I devices are of low risk, and are subject to little more than general controls and good manufacturing practices. Suction cups used in snake bite kits are an example of Class I devices. Class II devices additionally require special controls such as performance standards and/or restricted access. Hypodermic needles are an example of Class II devices. Class III devices additionally require pre-market approval (PMA) to legally enter the market. Pacemakers and life support equipment are examples of Class III devices.

New devices that have not been determined to have a pre-amendment equivalent are automatically placed in Class III. Medical devices that have not been submitted for classification are by default also relegated to Class III. With the exception of acupuncture needles (now in Class II), the traditional devices used by acupuncturists are Class III by default. Modern devices, such as lasers and electroacupuncture units, are often Class III not by default, but as a result of overt FDA determination processes.

To legally market Class I and Class II devices, manufacturers must submit a relatively simple 510k premarket notification. To market Class III devices, manufacturers must apply for and receive PMA. (21CFR860, 862-892) For PMA, devices must be demonstrated to the FDA's satisfaction as safe and effective for the intended uses and claimed indications. The FDA clears applications to market devices, and clears labeled claims and uses, but it does not strictly speaking 'approve' devices.

Prior to receiving PMA, investigational use of a Class III device is normally allowed to establish safety and efficacy. Investigators apply for an Investigational Device Exemption (IDE), which may be waived for non-significant risk device studies. Research on human subjects requires approval and oversight by an institutional review board (IRB), written informed consent, data collection and recordkeeping, among other strictures.(21CFR812) An overview of research requirements is on the FDA Internet website at: **http://www.fda.gov/oc/oha/toc.html** Purporting to do research, or prolonging a research project interminably, as a screen for treatment use of a device, is deemed 'commercialization of an IDE'. Commercialization of an IDE is illegal.

An investigational device is any Class III device that has not received PMA. (However, any device regardless of class, when used in an investigational protocol on human subjects, becomes an investigational device within the research context of use.) If a Class III device is used in a non-research treatment context, then the regulations governing research do not apply. The term 'investigational device' relates the FDA cleared use of a Class III device that lacks PMA. Cleared uses are not necessarily the only legal uses.

The cleared intended uses of a device are called the 'labeled uses'. All other medical uses are 'off-label uses'. Charging money for (i.e. commercializing) off-label uses is of questionable legality. There is a considerable gray area of regulatory authority here. In the absence of public health hazards, the FDA does not generally intercede in the off-label uses of cleared devices, leaving matters of medical practice to state medical boards. But if off-label medical claims for a device are advertised, that would be misbranding, and subject to FDA compliance action.

The treatment use (not in an investigational protocol) of a Class III device might be termed the 'off-label use of an un-labeled device'. As with off-label use of cleared devices, the FDA intercedes discretionarily into what is at times a regulatory gray area. It is illegal to commercially distribute Class III devices to providers for treatment use, and so possession of Class III devices may be subject to FDA confiscation. Class III devices for treatment are legally possessed when personally brought into the country from abroad, and when they are custom made devices. (21CFR812.3(b)) The provider encounters the same questionable legality of commercialization for off-label uses with Class III devices as with Class II devices, but probably a lower threshold of FDA response.

The FDA restricts Class III device promotion, medical claims and sales, sometimes invoking fraudulent use regulations. Fraudulent use is defined as promoting or selling devices that have 'not been scientifically proven safe and effective for such purposes', even if proceeding with good intentions. (FDA 1996a) In addition, the acupuncturist faces issues of malpractice liability, and (potentially) state regulatory body sanctions relating to standards of practice and scope of practice. Any willful violation of law would not be covered by malpractice insurance policies. Health insurance infrequently reimburses the treatment use of investigational devices.

If you choose to provide off-label uses of cleared devices, or to provide off-label uses of Class III un-labeled devices, then heed these four caveats:

1. Let use be visible only to your patients. Do not advertise, offer to the public at large, promote, nor commercialize your uses, and never overtly sell, lease or provide Class III devices (beyond clinical treatment use).

2. Document supportive evidence for your uses. Base use on evidence (which may include personal observations), proceeding in the belief that there are potential therapeutic benefits for specific medical conditions.

3. Inform patients in a written, signed consent process that the device and/or indications for the device are not FDA cleared.

Explicitly state that no safety and medical effectiveness claims are made for the device.

4. Provide use not in lieu of standards of care, but in addition to standards of care. Standards of care refers to both TOM standards and biomedical standards. The latter are enacted through timely and appropriate referrals.

In the medical mainstream, it is not rare to encounter off-label uses of devices and drugs cleared for marketing. However, it is uncommon to find the intentional treatment use of devices that have not been FDA cleared for marketing. Obtaining professional support for using an un-labeled device would likely prove difficult in any related negligence case. In contrast, TOM medical devices are predominantly not cleared for marketing. The acupuncturist's use of certain traditional yet un-labeled devices arguably could be supported by the standard practices of the profession and the provisions of state scope of practice laws and regulations.

The market reality is that Class III acupuncture devices are readily available to providers. The FDA has a longstanding compliance policy to ignore the sale of some (but not all) Class III acupuncture devices intended for treatment use. (FDA 1996b) In terms of legal realism, manufacturers, importers and distributors are at greater risk of compliance actions than circumspect individual providers.

There is a fundamental problem constituted by the Class III categorization of traditional devices used in moxibustion, cupping, coining and acupressure. It is not rectified by justifying use based on the acupuncture profession's standards, nor by residing in the FDA's discretion to ignore sales of Class III acupuncture devices. There is a shared moral obligation to seek FDA reclassification of Class III traditional acupuncture devices. A fair and expeditious process would go far in developing mutual respect and long term cooperation. The recent reclassification of needles is a first step in the right direction.

In the interim, implement a risk control strategy of substituting Class I and II devices for Class III devices whenever possible. This requires not just individual selection of substitute devices, but determinations from state acupuncture regulatory boards and professional associations that the substitute devices are within scope and suitable as a standard of practice. For example, if infrared lamps are to be used in indirect moxibustion, this should be formally considered by the state licensing body and acupuncture association, for acknowledgment as an acceptable practice. The process generates creditable legal support for practitioners, while marking distinct boundaries for the profession. Refer to California Association of Acupuncture & Oriental Medicine's model report on scope of practice. (1997 CAAOM)

Risk Control Strategies:
When using medical devices in a human subjects research context, strictly follow FDA rules for investigational protocols.

If you choose to provide off-label uses of cleared devices, or to provide off-label uses of Class III un-labeled devices:
    Let use be visible only to your patients.
    Base use on documented evidence.
    Inform patients in a written, signed consent process.
    Use in addition to TOM and biomedical standards of care.

Substitute Class I or II devices for Class III devices, as approved by state regulatory boards and professional associations.

Carefully note malpractice policy device and technique exclusions.

FDA Device Standards: Acupuncture Devices

Risks:
FDA regulatory compliance.

Discussion:
In 1996 the FDA reclassified acupuncture needles from Class III to Class II devices. Needles may be legally marketed to qualified practitioners for treatment use. Needles must be sterile and labeled for single use. (Fed.Register 1996)

Although acupuncture needles have been cleared for use in acupuncture practice, no medical indications for their use have been cleared. The intended use of needles as a tool in practice is the only labeled use. All claims of medical efficacy for the devices are off-label claims, and constitute mis-branding.

Searches of the FDA CDRH Product Code Classification Database (PCCD) have not produced any mention of traditional moxibustion, cupping, coining or acupressure devices. These physical medicine devices are Class III by default. Marketing is limited to investigational uses. They are not cleared for treatment use sales.

While traditional moxibustion devices (including herbal heating poultices) remain Class III, a number of alternative indirect moxibustion devices are rated Class I or II. These include moist heat, dry heat, chemical and electrical heat devices.

Most if not all electroacupuncture devices are Class III, including point locators, electro-diagnostic units, and electro-stimulator devices. Electroacupuncture devices are reviewed by the FDA as types of transcutaneous electrical nerve stimulators (TENS).

Historically, TENS units were adapted from electroacupuncture devices, and so we recognize an ironic situation.

Biostimulation lasers are all Class III devices. The use of biostimulation lasers for treatment constitutes off-label use of an unlabeled device, and is subject to previously mentioned restrictions. If one purchases a laser pointer pen and uses it for medical treatment, it is then considered to be a Class III medical device.

In addition to (and entirely separate from) medical device classification, lasers have an FDA hazard classification rated by power output. Lasers range from Class I to Class IV. Biostimulation lasers are usually Class IIIa or Class IIIb, and are defined as non-significant risk (NSR) devices.

Because biostimulation lasers are NSR devices, an investigational device exemption (IDE) is tacitly granted for investigational uses, without FDA notification. However, all other FDA requirements for research apply, including oversight by an IRB. (See FDA Device Standards - Background, above.)

Magnets are Class III when marketed for use as medical devices. In the absence of medical claims and intentions for use pursuant to sale, magnets are not medical devices at all. Magnetic jewelry, for instance, is just jewelry - unless it is labeled, promoted or advertised with claims of medical benefits.

To determine whether a specific device is cleared for marketing, ask the manufacturer for a copy of the clearance letter, or for the 510k or PMA number. Inquire at the CDRH (800) 638-2041, or by Internet: **http://www.fda.gov/cdrh/foicdrh.html**

Risk Control Strategies:
Ascertain FDA clearance, indications and class of your devices.

Refer to the risk control strategies of the previous section, and to the technical chapters for each type of acupuncture device.

FDA Standards: Herbs & Dietary Supplements

Risks:
Compliance with FDA regulations.

Discussion:
Herbal products and extracts, together with a range of supplements including vitamins, amino acids, enzymes and minerals, are regulated by the FDA as dietary supplements under the Dietary Supplement Health & Education Act of 1994 (DSHEA). A summary of the DSHEA is available on the Internet at **http://vm.cfsan.fda.gov/~dms/dietsupp.html** A brief review of key sections follows.

Labeling is one of the most important requirements of the DSHEA. Labels must explicitly identify the product as a dietary supplement. No medical claims may be made about a supplement's uses to diagnose, prevent, mitigate, treat, or cure a specific disease. If medical claims were made, the supplement would be considered an investigational new drug (IND). Ingredients (and quantities of each) must be listed on the label. The word 'dose' is not used because of medical connotations; 'serving size' is used instead.

The DSHEA defines a dietary supplement as adulterated if it presents 'a significant or unreasonable risk of illness or injury' when used as directed. Manufacturers (and compounders) are responsible for producing safe dietary supplements.

The DSHEA mandates that informational literature at retail outlets must offer a balanced view and not be misleading. Literature cannot promote a specific brand, and must not be displayed in immediate proximity with the supplements being sold.

A number of herbal products have been detained by the FDA. Enforcement actions identify misbranding, adulteration with controlled pharmaceuticals, and/or reports of consumer injury. A list of detained Chinese herbal medicine supplements is presented in FDA Import Alert#66-10, currently available on the Internet at **http://www.fda.gov/ora/fiars/ora_import_ia6610.html**.

Readers perusing the import alerts will realize that some seriously hazardous TOM herbal products have been detained. The FDA deserves our gratitude for enforcement actions which have removed unquestionably dangerous products from the market. Refer to Chapter 18 for more information on detained supplements.

Acupuncturists' provision of dietary supplements, herbal or otherwise, is also subject to: state scope of practice laws and regulations; state laws limiting the sale of certain herbs; and Fish & Wildlife Service regulation of endangered species parts. (Refer to Ch.18.)

Risk Control Strategies:
Check supplements offered for sale in your clinic for:
    DSHEA labeling compliance - remove if non-compliant.
    FDA Import Alert list - remove if listed.
    Ingredient safety - remove those with unsafe ingredients.

Make no claims of medical efficacy for supplements.

Immediately report adverse or unusual supplement side effects to the manufacturer and the FDA.

CHAPTER 13

TECHNICAL ASPECTS OF TREATMENT

The final context, Technical Aspects Of Treatment, is examined in detail over ten chapters. As the prelude, this chapter comments on the nature of the technical guidelines; defines 'Best Practices'; explains equipment sterilization & disinfection protocols; and closes with basic hygienic & safety practices.

The Nature Of The Technical Guidelines

Discussion:
This text does not attempt to present the full range of indications and contraindications for each acupuncture technique. Nor does it purport to give complete instruction in any TOM technique. It is assumed that the reader has obtained (or is in the process of obtaining) a comprehensive technical acupuncture education. The recommendations herein represent refinements of that training.

As it is not possible to foresee all practice conditions from afar, each acupuncturist must assess their own situation. They must also assess the adequacy of recommendations, and implement or improve upon them as they deem appropriate.

Not all of the techniques described are within the scope of practice of every acupuncturist. Risk control strategies and Best Practices, particularly those that recommend substitute devices, may or may not fall within current state definitions of scope of practice and standards of practice. Prior to implementation, confirm the approval of your state licensing board and professional association.

Best Practices

Discussion:
Best Practices are offered as well-reasoned, entirely implementable <u>minimum standards of practice</u> based on the ethical imperative to diminish harms. They are not 'best' in the sense of maximum standards, but best in the sense of being adequate for the control of several kinds of risk. Best Practices further convey the adaptation of acupuncture to the professional, legal and social contexts of American medicine.

Readers who find it necessary to substantially re-train themselves to adopt or improve Best Practice standards will be rewarded with the sense of security that comes from significant risk reduction and enhanced professional legitimacy. Best Practices often approximate practice standards required for inclusion in provider networks, HMO's, and other mainstream medical reimbursement and service venues.

Equipment Sterilization & Disinfection

Risks:
Bloodborne pathogen transmission.

Discussion:
The surest way to reduce equipment-related risks of bloodborne pathogen transmission is to exclusively use disposable critical instruments, and to promptly dispose of any blood or OPIM

contaminated instruments. The rationale for this strategy emerges from a discussion of equipment sterilization and decontamination.

To determine adequate equipment decontamination protocols, first consider the language of sterilization and disinfection as developed by the CDC. (CDC 1993) <u>Sterilization</u> kills all microbial life, including all bacterial endospores. <u>Disinfection</u> kills pathogenic microorganisms, but not all bacterial endospores.

Disinfection is rated at three levels: high, intermediate and low. <u>High level disinfection</u> kills all microorganisms and some bacterial spores, using an FDA-registered chemical sterilant solution. <u>Intermediate level disinfection</u> kills *mycobacterim tuberculosis var. bovis*, and weaker pathogens including Hepatitis B and HIV, using an EPA-registered tuberculocidal germicide solution, or a bleach solution. <u>Low level disinfection</u> kills some (but not all) viruses and bacteria using an EPA-registered chemical germicidal solution.

High level chemical disinfectants often contain glutaraldehyde, a chemical relative of formaldehyde. Glutaraldehyde is an airway irritant and skin irritant, and must be used with adequate ventilation such as an exhaust hood. Contaminated medical instruments require up to ten hours of exposure to the sterilant solution. High level disinfectant use requires very close adherence to manufacturer's instructions. Intermediate and low level disinfectants generally present less risk to the user.

However, ammonia based products (ammonia, quaternary ammonia compounds) should not be mixed with chlorine based products (bleach, sodium hypochlorite), as toxic gas is released.

The level of sterilization or disinfection required is determined by the uses of medical equipment. Instruments that penetrate tissue, or through which blood flows, are deemed <u>critical</u> instruments which require sterilization. Instruments that touch mucous membranes are defined as <u>semi-critical</u>, and require sterilization or high level disinfection. Instruments (and environmental surfaces) that only contact intact skin are defined as <u>non-critical</u>, and require intermediate level or low level disinfection.

By these definitions, acupuncture needles in all their forms are clearly critical instruments. If cupping cups draw blood or OPIM, that contamination might fit the 'blood flowing through' definition of critical instruments requiring sterilization. Yet without blood or OPIM contamination, cupping cups are non-critical instruments.

Coining (Gua Sha) friction devices can cause the extravasation of a small amount of blood. The quantity of blood is minute, yet the infective potential is not. Because scraped skin is not equivalent to intact skin, gua sha devices are at least semi-critical instruments.

While there are several methods of sterilizing critical equipment, each method presents a new set of risks. High level sterilant solutions are chemical hazards and are also subject to incorrect use. Autoclaving re-useable needles increases needlestick risks from additional needle handling. Incompletely cleaned needles, however well autoclaved, may still introduce foreign matter into patients. Autoclaves may malfunction in several ways, so documentation must be kept detailing maintenance and regular monitoring with biologic and thermal tests. The risk of breakage due to metal fatigue is greater for re-used needles. While re-useable needles can be processed properly, serious (and preventable) incidents of bloodborne pathogen infections have occurred. The exclusive use of pre-sterilized single use disposables controls these many risks. That policy honors the intent of the FDA requirement that needles be pre-sterilized and labeled as single use devices. (See Chapter 12.) Last but not least, the practice meets prevailing social and medical expectations of safe practice standards. Should there be any infection concerns, your critical equipment standards will be beyond reproach. The re-use of critical instruments is an invitation to harsh review in the event of a problem, because so many of the risks associated with re-usables are readily avoidable.

The cost of disposables is certainly not prohibitive to adopting them as the standard of practice. When the cost of the time spent cleaning needles is calculated, the use of disposables may well prove immediately economical. Long term economies arise from decreased risk of harm. The price of an acupuncture treatment should cover (or be adjusted to cover) the cost of disposable critical equipment and other disposable hygienic supplies.

The foregoing rationale supports:

> **1.** Exclusive use of pre-sterilized single-use needles, used once and immediately discarded after use into an approved sharps container. *This applies to every form of needle used in the practice of acupuncture.*
>
> **2.** Discarding of cupping cups that contact blood or OPIM, after careful disposal of their contents.
>
> **3.** Exclusive use of single-use disposable coining devices.

Refer to Chapters 14, 16 and 17 respectively for more information on these protocols.

Risk Control Strategies:
Use single use disposables for all critical, semi-critical, and blood or OPIM contacting instruments.

Hygienic & Safety Practices

Risks:

Disease transmission; failure to meet expectations of basic hygienic and safety practices.

Discussion:

Use disposable table paper to cover the treatment table, and a disposable paper pillow cover. Change table and pillow covers after each patient use. Fresh table paper offers a clean surface for the patient. The fresh pillow cover helps prevent transmission of lice. As an alternative, cotton sheets could be used to cover the table, and replaced after each use. Minimize handling of used linens (technically 'soiled' but not 'contaminated' unless contacting blood or OPIM), bag or otherwise contain them, and have them (preferably professionally) laundered with detergent and bleach. Similarly, gowns and draping materials should be disposables, or laundered with detergent and bleach before re-use.

Decontaminate treatment tables at the end of every shift, and whenever they become contaminated with blood or OPIM. Perform at least a low level decontamination before and after treatment of high risk patients. (See Ch. 6, Universal Precautions.) To perform intermediate level disinfection on smooth non-porous vinyl covered treatment tables:

* Wear as PPE rubberized heavy duty utility gloves.

* Remove visible contamination using a paper towel.

* Clean the surface with detergent and water.

* Wipe the surface with a liquid chemical germicide EPA registered as a tuberculocidal hospital disinfectant, or with a bleach solution. Follow manufacturer's instructions on the germicidal solution.

* Allow surface to air dry before use.

Similarly decontaminate sinks, work surfaces, and waste receptacles whenever they become contaminated with blood or OPIM, and on a regularly scheduled basis. (See Ch.6, Housekeeping.)

Decontaminate non-critical hand tools such as hemostats and forceps whenever they become contaminated with blood or OPIM, and at the end of every shift. Perform at least a low level decontamination before and after treatment of high risk patients. (See Ch. 6, Universal Precautions.) After washing, completely immerse hand tools in a decontaminant solution. Follow manufacturer's instructions on the germicidal solution. Bleach solutions corrode metals, especially aluminum. Regularly examine tools for corrosion, and replace damaged tools. Dispose of the decontaminant solution after use, pouring it down a drain without splashing.

Suitable intermediate level decontaminant solutions can be made from household bleach. Effective ratios of bleach to water are between **1:10** and **1:100**. The stronger concentrations are more appropriate for porous surfaces. Bleach solutions must be made fresh daily and stored in a dated and labeled container. Alcohol evaporates too quickly for adequate contact time, and is not recommended for disinfecting environmental surfaces. (MMWR 1993)

Lysol® is an example of a low level decontaminant solution.

Risk Control Strategies:
Use fresh treatment table coverings, gowns and drapes for each patient.

Decontaminate treatment tables whenever they become contaminated with blood or OPIM, and at the end of every shift. Perform at least low level decontamination before and after treatment of high risk patients. (See Chapter 6, Universal Precautions.)

Decontaminate sinks, work surfaces, and waste receptacles whenever they become contaminated with blood or OPIM, and on a regularly scheduled basis.

Decontaminate non-critical hand tools such as hemostats and forceps whenever they become contaminated with blood or OPIM, and at the end of every shift. Perform at least low level decontamination before and after treatment of high risk patients. (See Chapter 6, Universal Precautions.)

CHAPTER 14

ACUPUNCTURE NEEDLES

In the technical aspect of Acupuncture Needles we address accountability for needles; bloodborne pathogen risks; potentials for structural harm; needle manufacturing flaws; and requirements for a travel kit.

Accountability For Needles

Risks:
Loss of control over needles prior to proper disposal.

Discussion:
Acupuncturists are legally accountable for every acupuncture needle that enters their premises. They remain accountable until contaminated needles are properly contained and transferred to a licensed regulated medical waste disposal company in the manner described by federal, state and local regulations.

Patients occasionally request a sample needle to show friends and family. If the provider complies with that request, they have lost control over the use and disposal of the needle, and yet remain legally accountable for that professional tool. The provider is liable for whatever personal harm may result.

This raises legitimate concerns about all types of retained needles. For example, consider the problem with ear press needles. These miniature 'tacks' are inserted and taped to ear points, and left in place for up to a week. Yet the tape often fails to hold them in place. They fall out and are frequently unaccounted for. Is an ear press needle long enough to transmit disease? *Absolutely.* The lost ear press needle that is stepped on barefoot by another person, or rolled on in the bedding, may deliver deadly infective harm.

Additionally, retained needles pose a greater infection risk than non-retained needles. Infections in the cartilage of the ear are particularly difficult to treat, and can lead in the worst cases to the loss of the outer ear, or to bacterial endocarditis. (Davis & Powell 1985; Lee & McIlwain 1985; Gilbert 1987; Sorensen 1990)

Use taped seeds in place of press needles and other types of retained needles.

Risk Control Strategies:
Never give needles to patients for self-treatment or as samples.

Substitute taped seeds for ear press needles and other types of retained needles.

Ascertain local and state regulated waste disposal requirements.

Keep records of needle disposal through a licensed regulated medical waste disposal company.

Bloodborne Pathogens

Risks:
Bloodborne pathogen transmission.

Discussion:
Handwashing is an efficacious work practice to prevent disease transmission. Wash hands before inserting needles, between each different patient contact, after removing gloves, and immediately after any blood or OPIM exposure. (See Chapter 6.)

Only use pre-sterilized single use disposable needles. This applies to acupuncture needles of every type, from filiform to prismatic to seven star needles. (See Chapter 13.) The medical literature reports several HBV outbreaks related to re-usable acupuncture needles. (Stryker et al 1986; Kent et al 1988; Slater et al 1988; CDR Weekly 1992)

Use needles only once, and directly dispose into a sharps container after use. The re-use of needles designed (or labeled) for single use circumvents the many advantages of disposables, and introduces a remarkable liability should such needles fail in use. Imagine how an attorney might question your judgment to re-use an inexpensive device labeled for single use. Re-use of disposables is a false economy.

Use needles that are singly packaged. Bulk pack needles suffer longer air exposure time after the package is initially opened and before the last needles are used, leading to compromised needle sterility at time of use. Handling of adjacent needles in the package also jeopardizes sterility.

The acupuncturist encounters risks of blood exposure associated with needling. These risks are primarily from bloodletting techniques; during needle removal; and from needlestick injuries.

<u>Bloodletting techniques</u> are performed with a disposable lancet, with the intent of removing several drops of blood. Glove both hands prior to performing this technique, because blood is certain

to be produced. Have one or more cotton balls at the ready to absorb the small amount of blood. Unless saturated with blood, the cotton balls are disposable as contaminated waste. If gloves become contaminated by blood during the procedure, remove and discard them, wash hands, and re-glove to complete the procedure.

On the <u>removal of filiform acupuncture needles</u>, as many as one point in five might bleed a droplet or two. The usual response is to apply pressure to those points with a cotton ball. At a minimum, glove the hand that holds the cotton ball, while removing needles with the other hand. The risk control advantages are these: when repositioning the cotton ball, blood on the cotton ball might only contact the provider's glove, and not the provider's skin. If the acupuncturist attempts to apply pressure, but their gloved hand misses or slides off the bleeding site, only the glove is likely to contact blood. Because gloving is not necessary until needle removal, no loss of needling dexterity occurs. Keep a box of PPE gloves on the supply table. Very little time is needed to don a glove.

Is gloving for needle removal mandated by OSHA? OSHA requires PPE for exposure risks remaining after engineering and work practice controls have been implemented. OSHA notes that gloves may not be required if hand contact with blood is not anticipated. The question revolves around the likelihood of exposure. A careful practitioner may in fact rarely contact blood on needle removal and pressure application. Given the risks and costs of an exposure incident, is 'rarely' good enough for you and for your employees?

OSHA offers the work practice of having the patient apply pressure with a cotton ball to their own injection site, as a way of preventing provider exposure to blood without using gloves. But needles are placed at several sites simultaneously in acupuncture, and more than one may bleed, rendering this solution impractical.

When a greater margin of safety can be provided so readily, a lesser standard of practice is difficult to support. If the question of regulatory mandate is at all equivocal, its pragmatic resolution is not. At a minimum, glove the hand that holds the cotton ball while needles are being removed with the other hand. After glove removal, dispose of the gloves as contaminated waste and then wash your hands.

<u>Contaminated needlestick injuries</u> are very serious exposure incidents. (Refer to Chapter 6.) Prevention requires constant vigilance on the part of the acupuncturist. Locate red plastic sharps containers in close proximity to every treatment table. Sharps containers must be fastened to a wall or securely taped to a horizontal surface, to prevent being knocked over and risk having the contents spill out. Replace the containers when no more than two thirds full, to prevent incomplete containment or deflection of deposited needles. Deposit used needles directly from the patient into the sharps container, with no secondary collection tray. This minimizes handling, and thereby decreases needlestick risk.

Record a needle count after needle insertion, and tabulate a count on needle removal, to be certain that all needles are removed and accounted for. If a needle accidentally falls out prior to the intentional removal of it, the count at removal will be off, and the acupuncturist will be alerted to locate the missing needle. This work practice helps prevent needlestick injuries, as well as potential harm from accidentally retained needles.

When several procedures are planned, order them in such a way as to minimize blood exposure risks. For example, if both cupping and needling are planned for a single acupuncture point, cup first and needle second. This will draw less blood than when done in the reverse order. (Refer to Chapters 16 and 17.)

For finer points of site preparation and needle handling, refer to Clean Needle Technique Manual For Acupuncturists. (NAF 1997)

There are occasional reports of acupuncturists needling patients through articles of clothing. In the bitter cold of Chinese winters, this reputedly was a common traditional practice. Irrespective of whether it increases infection risks, the practice is socially unacceptable in America. It creates the appearance (and testifies to the fact) of sub-standard care. Do not consider needling patients through articles of clothing. Have patients disrobe sufficiently to expose needling sites.

Risk Control Strategies:

Wash hands before needle insertion, between each patient contact, after removing gloves, and immediately after any blood or OPIM exposure.

Use only pre-sterilized single-use one-per-packet disposable needles. Use needles only once and directly discard in sharps container.

On needle removal, at a minimum, glove the hand holding the cotton ball.

Glove both hands for bloodletting at points.

Locate red plastic sharps containers in close proximity to every treatment table, and secure them to a wall or horizontal surface.

Replace sharps containers when no more than two thirds full.

Record needle count after needle insertion and on needle removal.

Plan order of interventions to minimize blood exposure.

Do not needle patients through articles of clothing.

Carry professional liability insurance.

Structural Damage

Risks:
Nerve, organ or arterial damage from needles.

Discussion:
Basic technical training in acupuncture addresses the prevention of needle damage to bodily structures. The following comments reinforce and focus that training.

Whenever practical, position patients for treatment so that they are reclined, supine, or prone. When needling a seated patient, be in constant attendance, elicit verbal feedback, and maintain visual assessment. (See Chapter 9.) Place a sturdy stepstool by each treatment table to assist patients.

Cases of nerve injury have been reported involving the needling of points over small nerves in the region from the elbow to the fingers. When needling points such as SI 8, Ht 3 or Ht 7, use very fine gauge needles (e.g. Japanese #1-3), and a delicate approach to obtain light stimulus, foregoing any further needle manipulation. These precautions will minimize physical trauma to fine nerves.

There may be risk of spinal nerve injury when needling lower Du meridian points in the presence of occult spinal bifida. While unaware of injury cases to date, the potential for injury is noteworthy.

The most reported organ injury is to the lungs. (Huet et al 1990; Gray et al 1991; Devouassoux et al 1994; Norheim 1994; Norheim & Fonnebo 1995) Pneumothaces have been caused by needles at Lv 14 and GB 21, among other points over the lung area. Horizontal needle placement (as at Lv 14) and oblique needle placement (as at GB 21) can decrease vertical depth of penetration and provide a margin of safety for points over the lungs.

To prevent needling an artery, prepare and refer to a list of points near or over arteries. Point palpation prior to needling can disclose the presence of an artery.

Certain acupuncture points entail higher risks of structural harm. Alternate point selections should be considered when possible. Prepare and refer to a list of 'higher risk' points and alternate point selections with similar energetics. If choosing higher risk points, use impeccable point location, shallow and brief insertions, and little if any needle manipulation. Higher risk points include:

Ren 22	TW 17	UB 1
St 1	St 9	St 12

Do not needle acupuncture points inside the orbital cavity unless directly supervised or extensively trained by a specialist in those points.

When Qi cannot be obtained at a conservative needle depth, let the needle rest and allow Qi to come to the needle over time. It is not worth obtaining Qi at the risk of damaging organs.

Gauging proper needle depth and location on grossly obese patients is particularly difficult. Accept this limitation as a fact of life, and not as a reflection on your skill. If there is error, let it be on the side of safety. A cross-sectional anatomic atlas is a valuable reference. (Holland 1989)

An imbedded needle technique called *okibari* is used in Japan. It involves clipping the handle off a short horizontally inserted needle, leaving a needle fragment permanently implanted under the skin. Fragments have been identified on x-ray at some distance from the site of original insertion, and in their migrations have caused serious medical harm. Imbedded needles are intrinsically hazardous, and should never be used. (Galutin & Autin 1988; Hasegawa et al 1990; Murata et al 1990; Sakai et al 1994)

Needle breakage is rare, but complications from several have been reported in the medical literature. (Southworth & Hartwig 1990; Gi et al 1994) Stable positioning of patients, a delicate hand on needle insertions, and single-use needles serve to control this risk.

Point injection therapy (aquapuncture) uses hypodermic needles to inject acupuncture points with normal saline or other solutions. Not all states define this practice as being within the legal scope of acupuncture. Those that do may explicitly list permissible injection substances. The practitioner should possess training in hypodermic needling and be aware of nerve damage potential from the needle's beveled cutting edge. Allergic reactions to normal saline injection are uncommon but possible, and probably related to the solution's preservatives. Other solutions present greater allergic response risks. Be prepared to respond to anaphylactic shock. (Refer to Chapter 9.)

Risk Control Strategies:
Whenever practical, position patients in a reclined, supine or prone position.

When needling a seated patient, be in constant attendance, elicit verbal feedback, and maintain visual assessment.

Minimize physical trauma to fine nerves of the forearms and hands through use of thin needles, a delicate approach and minimal needle manipulation.

For points over the lungs, consider horizontal and oblique needle placements to decrease vertical depth of penetration.

Prepare and refer to a list of points near or over arteries.

Prepare and refer to a list of 'higher risk' points and alternate point selections with similar energetics.

Never use imbedded needles.

Err on the side of caution.

Manufacturing Flaws

Risks:
Needle manufacturing flaws.

Discussion:
Acupuncturists have shared the following three examples of flawed needles. The accounts are presented in support of a needle inspection protocol.

Some years ago, batches of one Chinese brand of pre-sterilized disposable needles appeared to be contaminated with machine oil. Acupuncturists using the needles reported a small dark spot

Ch.14 Acupuncture Needles 169

remained at sites of insertion. This may have been a droplet of machine oil left under the skin.

A set of un-sterilized gold acupuncture needles was autoclaved. Thereafter, gold plating flaked off when the needles were flexed.

In ten years of experience with one brand of single-use disposable needles, an acupuncturist experienced two instances of handle detachment after insertion, making needle removal challenging.

Acupuncturists are extraordinarily dependent on the quality of acupuncture needles. To control risks associated with manufacturing flaws, perform and document an assessment on a small sample of sterile needles from each new shipment:

* Note integrity of sealed packaging.

* Note straightness of needles inside packaging - no bent needles.

* Assess frank contamination - test by twirling several needles on white absorbent paper. No mark should be left.

* Assess under magnification for smoothness of shaft and point - use 15-30x magnifying lens.

* Assess for burrs or hooks on point - test by inserting needles into a cotton ball and pulling them back out. No fibers should be hooked.

* Assess handle attachment - test by twisting handle and tugging on shaft. No separation or loosening should occur.

Discard test needles in a sharps container.

Call the manufacturer and supplier immediately about needles failing inspection, or failing in clinical use. Follow up with written letters, and keep copies for your files. This vital information could lead to the recall of defective products, and could thereby protect other acupuncturists and their patients. If response is in any way inadequate to the assessment or control of a hazard, contact the FDA. Inspect your stock of needles and remove those from the same batch as a flawed needle, so that patients will be protected.

While needle manufacturing flaws are rare events, these simple precautions add a margin of safety.

Risk Control Strategies:
Document inspection of needle samples from every new shipment.

Call and write manufacturer and supplier immediately about needles failing inspection or failing in clinical use. If response is inadequate, contact the FDA.

Remove from stock needles in the same batch as a flawed needle.

Travel Kit Requirements

Risks:
Travel kit safety and regulatory compliance.

Discussion:
Assess the travel kit, which accompanies the acupuncturist on outcalls, for safety and regulatory compliance. Several key provisions follow.

Ch.14 Acupuncture Needles

Transport pre-sterilized needles in such a way that they do not get bent or poke through their packaging. Their package edges should be protected from becoming dog-eared and accidentally flexed open. A plastic 3x5 file card box with a hinged latching lid protects sterile packaged needles in transport.

Protect disposable exam gloves from puncture damage in transport. Another plastic 3x5 file card box serves to house gloves.

For the disposal of used needles, bring a pint-sized red plastic sharps container. Disposal of needles directly into this type of container reduces risk by preventing the re-handling of contaminated needles that would be required if they were first placed in another type of container for transport. OSHA requires that sharps containers must be transported in a way that secures them in an upright position at all times. This is accomplished by taping the sharps container very securely to a metal tray. Place the tray on a flat surface with clear access, near to where you are working. Open the sharps container just prior to needle removal, place contaminated needles in it, and then close it immediately thereafter, to minimize the risk of an accidental spill.

Do not transport or use a sharps container placed inside a portable 'doctors black bag' or any other type of case which carries your equipment. You will not have clear lines of sight and access, and may not even notice dropping a contaminated needle into the recesses of the bag, where it could easily be hidden among other equipment and pose a needlestick injury risk.

Given that anti-bacterial soap may not be available at a housecall, wash hands with available soap and water, and then use an anti-microbial hand sanitizer (e.g. Hibistat® germicidal handwipe; AlCare® emollimented alcohol foam spray; Purell® hand sanitizer).

Risk Control Strategies:
Transport sterile needles in a protective container.

Transport disposable gloves in a protective container.

Transport contaminated needles in a closed red plastic sharps container taped securely to a tray and kept upright.

When anti-bacterial soap is not available, use plain soap and water, followed by use of an anti-bacterial hand sanitizer.

BEST PRACTICES

ACUPUNCTURE NEEDLES

Never give needles to patients for self-treatment or as samples.

Substitute taped seeds for ear press needles and indwelling needles.

Keep records of needle disposal through a licensed regulated medical waste disposal company.

Wash hands before needle insertion, between each patient contact, after removing gloves, and immediately after any blood or OPIM exposure.

Use only pre-sterilized single-use one-per-packet disposable needles. Use needles only once and discard in sharps container directly.

On needle removal, at a minimum, glove the hand holding the cotton ball while the other hand removes the needles.

Glove both hands for minor bloodletting procedures.

Locate red plastic sharps containers in close proximity to every treatment table, and secure them to a wall or horizontal surface.

Replace sharps containers when two thirds full.

Record needle count after insertion and on needle removal.

Plan order of interventions to minimize blood exposure (e.g. cup before needling).

Do not needle patients through their clothing.

Whenever practical, position patients in a reclined, supine or prone position.

When needling a seated patient, be in constant attendance, elicit verbal feedback, and maintain visual assessment.

Minimize physical trauma to fine nerves of the forearms and hands through use of thin needles, a delicate approach and minimal needle manipulation.

For points over the lungs, consider horizontal and oblique needle placements to decrease vertical depth of penetration.

Prepare and refer to a list of points near or over arteries.

Prepare and refer to a list of 'higher risk' points and alternate point selections with similar energetics.

Never use imbedded needles.

Err on the side of caution.

Document inspection of a needle sample from every new shipment.

Call and write manufacturer and supplier immediately about needles failing inspection or failing in clinical use. If response is inadequate, contact the FDA.

Remove from stock all needles in the same batch as a flawed needle.

Travel kit: Transport sterile needles in a protective container.

Travel kit: Transport disposable gloves in a protective container.

Travel kit: Transport contaminated needles in a closed red plastic sharps container taped securely to a tray.

Outcalls: When anti-bacterial soap is not available, use plain soap and water, followed by use of an anti-bacterial hand sanitizer.

Carry professional liability insurance.

CHAPTER 15

MOXIBUSTION

In the technical aspect of Moxibustion we first examine indirect moxibustion, identifying and controlling smoke & fire risks, and potentials for accidental burns. Direct moxibustion topics include technical notes; biomedical contraindications; and mis-attribution to abuse. The chapter closes with regulatory compliance issues.

Indirect Moxibustion: Smoke & Fire

Risks:
Smoke nuisance; smoke detector activation; fires.

Discussion:
Traditional indirect moxibustion burns 'moxa wool' to warm acupuncture points or larger areas. This practice presents smoke nuisance, smoke detector activation and fire risks.

The fumes of burning moxa wool generate a distinct smoke nuisance. New patients and neighboring tenants wonder if illicit substances are being smoked. Employees complain of the smell. Some individuals report headaches from moxa fumes.

The accidental activation of smoke detectors is not necessarily a minor inconvenience, but a potential hazard in its own right. Imagine patients in several treatment areas, somewhat disrobed and with needles inserted, reacting to the alarm in panic. The possibilities for injuries are notable. Consider as well the alarm's effects on occupants of adjacent offices.

Smoke detectors provide early warning of fire, and clearly protect life and property. De-activation of smoke detectors is not a defensible action.

Indirect moxibustion <u>fire risks</u> come from accidental contact of a moxa pole with flammable material, hot ashes falling, incomplete extinguishing, and overheating of moxa pole holders. A moxa pole holder is a small hollowed metal cylinder, closed on the base, designed to have a moxa pole vertically inserted with the pole's ember tip placed down into the recess of the holder. The holder is intended to extinguish the moxa pole, but it may not do so quickly. Over the course of a day, moxa pole holders can get hot enough to scorch a wooden table top.

As substitutes for burning moxa wool, consider the following options. Moist heat devices include hydrocollators, which contain and warm water for the immersion of heat packs. Chemical dry heat devices come in sealed packets. Air exposure or compression of a packet initiates an exothermic reaction. A simple dry heat device consists of a small flannel sack loosely filled with flax seeds and sewn closed, heated a minute or so in a microwave oven. Electrical dry heat devices include infra-red lamps, a commonly used substitute.

Infra-red lamps present a different but favorable set of risks when compared with moxa wool devices. Heat lamps can tip over, and must have stable, heavy bases. The lamp's heat element should be partially enclosed by a protective housing. Care must be taken to position lamps to prevent accidental burns or contact with flammable materials.

The elemental appeal of live embers and herbs is well appreciated. Yet in decades of clinical experience the author has seen no marked superiority in the therapeutic effects of traditional moxa wool devices, as compared with alternative heat sources.

Before initiating use of a substitute device, ascertain approval by your state regulatory board and professional association. Traditional moxibustion devices are FDA Class III. It is preferable to obtain Class II or Class I substitute indirect moxibustion devices.

Risk Control Strategies:
Use substitute heat sources for indirect moxibustion (moist heat, dry heat, infra-red lamps).

Indirect Moxibustion: Accidental Burns

Risks:
Accidental skin burns.

Discussion:
Given the potential for most forms of indirect moxa to accidentally cause burns, careful technique is required. Do not give patients moxa poles for self treatment. While well intended, this practice extends your liability into circumstances over which you have no control. It is also constitutes an overt sale of a Class III device.

Indirect moxibustion is contraindicated on patients who are unable to sense heat and pain. The neurologic damage of diabetes can produce these sensory deficits. Patients could easily sustain unintended burns.

When burning moxa wool on the handle of an inserted needle, first slide a square of aluminum foil over the needle to act as an ash catcher. Use a metal-handled needle. Do not burn loosely bundled unsupported moxa wool on a needle handle, as embers may easily fall off. Instead, cut a short section of a thin moxa roll to place on the needle handle. Remove the moxa roll before it is entirely burned, to reduce the risk of hot ash fall. As an alternative to a section of moxa roll, moxa wool may be pressed into a metal needle cap, which is then fitted onto a metal Japanese-style needle handle.

Certain traditional indirect moxibustion techniques present conspicuous risks for accidental burns. One technique is next described in detail, as an example of needless risk.

A paper towel is soaked in a warming oil, and then placed on a patient's back. The edges of the paper towel are folded up to form a rim. Loose moxa wool is scattered over the towel, and the moxa wool is ignited. Much smoke is produced. When the oil-soaked paper towel covered with burning moxa wool embers becomes uncomfortably hot, it is removed. However, removing it is no mean feat. If the paper towel sags at an edge, hot embers will fall out. If the sodden paper towel is pulled too taut in an effort to support the edges, it will tear and hot embers will fall. Add to that the risk that the moxa wool will ignite the paper towel.

With a modicum of ingenuity, equivalent yet far safer therapeutic heat applications can be designed using substitute devices.

Risk Control Strategies:
Do not give patients moxa wool or moxa poles for self treatment.

For moxa on the handle of an inserted needle:
    use a metal-handled needle.
     place a foil ash catcher around the base of the needle.

use sections of moxa roll, removed before entirely burned, or use needle caps with moxa wool pressed into them.

Use alternatives to high burn risk indirect moxibustion techniques.

Direct Moxibustion: Technical Notes

Risks:
Fire; unintended burns; use of moxibustion restricted points.

Discussion:
Direct moxibustion intentionally generates small (~5mm diameter) second or third degree burns at acupuncture points, traditionally using small cones of compressed moxa wool as the heat source. The cones are ignited with an incense stick.

There is a fire risk, but moxa cones are small enough to be extinguished between the thumb and forefinger. It is prudent to have a small cup of water at hand during the procedure. In contrast to indirect moxibustion, relatively little smoke is produced.

If ignited moxa cones fall off, unintended burns can result. To prevent moxa cones from falling off, position the patient appropriately, and secure the cone to the skin with a thin slip of petroleum jelly (or an adherent designed for moxa cones). A slip of saliva is not an acceptable adherent. Do not blow on the cones too hard, in hastening their burning, as they may become dislodged.

Attaining proficiency in the art of direct moxibustion requires specific training. The technique should not be attempted without that training. The tradition of direct moxibustion is marginally represented in the modern Chinese synthesis of TOM. A more extensive review of applications and point restrictions comes through the pre-war teachings of Cheng Tan An, carried in the work of James Tin Yao So. (So, 1977) Consult this source for a comprehensive list of direct moxibustion point restrictions.

Observe and chart the condition of the moxibustion site as healing progresses. Chart the lack of significant findings, if healing is progressing normally. Preventively apply an antiseptic to the burn site (e.g. Betadine®) after treatment.

Risk Control Strategies:
Develop and refer to a list of points with direct moxibustion restrictions.

Keep a cup of water at hand during direct moxibustion treatments.

To prevent moxa cones from falling off, position the patient appropriately, and secure cones with a thin slip of petroleum jelly (or an adherent designed for moxa cones).

Chart follow-up observations including normal healing.

Preventively apply an antiseptic after direct moxibustion treatment.

Direct Moxibustion: Biomedical Contraindications

Risks:
Biomedical contraindications.

Discussion:
Direct moxibustion is contraindicated in the presence of certain biomedical conditions. Diabetics frequently have poor micro-

circulation and exhibit difficulty in wound healing. This problem is pronounced on the feet, where the non-healing of a minor wound can lead to sepsis and amputation. Significant burn healing risks are also present in immuno-compromised patients.

Patients with a history of keloid scar formation risk unsightly raised scars. Facial points are also contraindicated for cosmetic reasons. Infants and small children are not candidates for this technique.

The quantity and location of direct moxibustion is restricted in pregnancy. Direct moxibustion is also usually contraindicated in patients with high blood pressure.

Risk Control Strategies:
Do not use direct moxibustion on patients with seriously impaired immune systems; patients with a history of keloid scar formation; and on infants or small children. Do not use facial points.

Use direct moxibustion with caution in pregnancy, high blood pressure, and diabetes. Never use direct moxa on feet of diabetics.

Direct Moxibustion: Mis-Attribution

Risks:
Mis-attribution of direct moxa burns to abuse.

Discussion:
The burns or scars of direct moxibustion can be mis-attributed to abuse, particularly on minors. Make patients aware of the need to educate family members and other care providers. Provide patients with handout materials describing direct moxibustion.

Use written, signed informed consent for moxibustion. Refer to Informed Consent in Chapter 8, and to FDA status in Chapter 12.

Risk Control Strategies:
Provide patients with handout materials describing direct moxibustion and its sequelae.

Let patients know the importance of their educational outreach to family members and other caregivers.

Obtain written, signed informed consent for moxibustion.

Regulatory Compliance

Risks:
Compliance with regulatory requirements.

Discussion:
First ascertain whether the use of moxibustion is within your legal scope of practice. Then assess and document your training in moxibustion, prior to including it in your clinical repertoire.

Traditional moxibustion devices are FDA Class III, not cleared for marketing. If you choose to use traditional moxibustion devices for treatment, implement the Class III device caveats from Chapter 12.

Risk Control Strategies:
Use moxibustion only if within your scope, training and competency.

If you choose to use traditional moxibustion devices for treatment, implement the Class III device caveats from Chapter 12.

BEST PRACTICES

MOXIBUSTION

Use substitute heat sources for indirect moxibustion (moist heat, dry heat, infra-red lamps).

Do not give patients moxa or moxa poles for self treatment.

Indirect moxibustion is contraindicated on:
* *patients unable to detect heat or pain.*

For moxa on the handle of an inserted needle:
use a metal-handled needle.
place foil ash catcher around the base of the needle.
use sections of moxa pole, removed before entirely burned, or use needle caps with moxa wool pressed into them.

Use alternatives to high burn risk indirect moxibustion techniques.

Develop and refer to a list of direct moxa point restrictions.

Keep water at hand during direct moxibustion treatments.

To prevent moxa cones from falling off, position the patient appropriately, and secure cones with a thin slip of petroleum jelly (or adherent designed for moxa cones).

Chart follow-up observations including normal healing.

Preventively apply an antiseptic after direct moxibustion.

Direct moxibustion is contraindicated on:
* *the feet of diabetics*
* *patients with impaired immune systems*
* *patients with keloid scar formation history*
* *infants and small children*
* *facial points*

Direct moxibustion is used with caution in:
* *pregnancy*
* *high blood pressure*
* *diabetes*

Provide patients with handout materials describing direct moxibustion and its sequelae.

Let patients know the importance of their educational outreach to family members and other caregivers.

Obtain written, signed informed consent for moxibustion.

If you choose to use traditional moxibustion devices for treatment, apply Class III device caveats from Chaper 12.

CHAPTER 16

CUPPING

The technical aspect of Cupping opens with technical notes which identify and suggest controls for fire & burn risks and excessive pressure risks. We then develop work practices and PPE protocols to control bloodborne pathogen risks. The chapter closes with discussion of regulatory compliance.

Technical Notes

Risks:
Fire & burn risks from flame-induced vacuum techniques; fluid filled blisters from excessive pressure; contraindicated uses.

Discussion:
Flame-induced vacuum techniques can - and indeed have - caused fires and accidental burns leading to malpractice suits. One technique involves wrapping a small coin in an alcohol-soaked cotton ball, which is then placed in the cup and ignited to create a vacuum. With rapid and secure placement of the cup on the skin, no additional oxygen is available and the flame dies. However, the flaming cotton and hot coin may fall onto the patient's skin, or onto their clothing.

Another technique uses a hemostat to grip an alcohol soaked cotton ball, which is ignited, held in the cup momentarily, and then removed as the cup is swiftly placed on the skin. While probably safer than the coin technique, close attention must be paid to the amount of alcohol used on the cotton ball. Too much alcohol and a swift motion in removing the flaming cotton ball causes a stream of burning alcohol to be ejected from the cotton ball.

The fire and burn risks of flame-induced vacuum cups are controlled by substituting pump-induced vacuum cups.

Skin becomes thinner and weaker with advancing age. Prolonged cortisone use can also produce this effect in younger individuals. In this condition, (and also on very damp bodies) it is relatively easy for the suction of cupping to create large blood or fluid filled blisters, which then may become infected after breaking. Patients with bleeding disorders, and those on anti-coagulant medications, are not good candidates for cupping. Do not cup over non-intact skin areas.

The use of pump-induced vacuum cups allows for very careful regulation of suction pressure, a key to preventing blister formation.

Cups with clear walls enable the acupuncturist to observe the presence, location and quantity of any suctioned blood or OPIM. Bamboo cups and opaque plastic cups do not meet this condition.

Cupping produces circular dark purplish 'bruise' marks which gradually resolve over several days. Inform patients about the appearance, and provide educational handout materials so that they can educate family members and other caregivers. Use signed written informed consent for cupping, as it uses Class III devices.

Risk Control Strategies:
Use only clear-walled pump-induced vacuum cups.

Do not use fire-induced vacuum cups.

Cupping contraindications:
* frail elderly   * chronic cortisone users
* bleeding disorders   * anti-coagulant medications
* over non-intact skin areas

Adjust pressure to avoid causing blood or fluid filled blisters.

Inform patients about cupping marks and provide educational handout materials.

Obtain signed written informed consent for cupping.

Bloodborne Pathogens

Risks:
Bloodborne pathogen risks from drawing blood or OPIM into cups.

Discussion:
Glove both hands for all cupping techniques, as there is always the possibility of drawing blood or OPIM, whether intended or not. If cups become contaminated with blood or OPIM, they have the potential to transmit disease. Do not re-use blood or OPIM contaminated cups. Avoid or minimize blood removal by cupping. The rationales and work practices for these stipulations follow.

If a site is to be needled and cupped in the same treatment, cup first and then needle afterwards. Blood is less likely to be drawn this way, reducing contamination of cups and exposure risks of acupuncturists.

Blood may enter the valve of a pump-induced vacuum cup if the cup is positioned to allow such drainage, or if enough blood accumulates in the cup irrespective of the cup's positioning. If the valve stem is bent or pressed to the side, it will leak. Subsequent cleaning of the valve is problematic. Containment and decontamination problems render pump-induced vacuum cups with a 40-50mm diameter at the base (2-4 ounce capacity) unsuitable for drawing a quantity of blood over 1.5 teaspoons (7.5 ml). Smaller cups are only suitable for trace blood containment without valve contamination. If it is anticipated that blood exposure to the valve cannot be prevented, then do not cup.

Cups eventually lose suction and fall off the patient's body. Provide continuous hand support (both hands gloved) to all cups that are drawing blood, to prevent cups falling off when they lose suction.

When cupping a site just previously needled, or over an inserted needle, one is likely to draw a small amount (~1 teaspoonful, ~5ml) of blood into the suction cup. Position pump-induced vacuum cups to avoid blood entering the valve area. Use cups that are at least 40mm diameter at the base (2-3 ounce capacity). Glove both hands and have paper toweling ready to absorb the small quantity of blood. Break the seal between the cup and skin gently, in an area on the rim where there is no blood or where there is the least likelihood of blood leakage. Absorb the blood with paper toweling, pack the inner surface of the cup with a paper towel, and dispose of cup and towels as contaminated waste in a plastic bag lined trash can. If the paper towel is saturated with blood, such that it might leak or release blood if compressed, then it must be disposed of as regulated waste. In that case, place it in a red plastic bag, seal the bag, and store for transfer to a regulated waste disposal company. Remove and dispose of contaminated gloves (red bag if gloves are bloody) and wash hands. Then re-glove if further contact with the cupped area, or other exposures, are expected.

Ch.16 Cupping 191

If intending to draw more than a teaspoonful (~5ml) of blood, repeat the above procedure, drawing no more than ~5ml into a cup at one time. As an alternative to absorbing the cup's contents on paper toweling, the contents might be emptied down a closely situated sink drain and the cup carefully rinsed, taking care to avoid any splashing. Decontaminate the sink following protocols in Ch. 13.

Whenever a blood or OPIM splash hazard is present, supply and have all employees at risk use lab coats and face shields as PPE in addition to gloves.

The decontamination of cupping devices presents many challenges, given that they are not designed to be steam or dry heat sterilized. Bamboo cups used with a hot-water-induced vacuum technique may crack in an autoclave, and their hot water bath is insufficient to sterilize them. Glass cups used with flame-induced vacuum techniques are not made from tempered glass, and may explode in an autoclave. Glass and plastic cups with pump-induced vacuums have a rubber valve housing which would be destroyed by autoclaving. Chemical sterilants present potential glutaraldehyde exposure and error in use risks. The resolution of the problem is to treat blood or OPIM contaminated cups as disposable items. (See Ch. 13, Equipment Sterilization & Disinfection.)

Cups, when used over intact skin and not contacting blood or OPIM, fit the definition of non-critical instruments. Presumably the pressure of the cup edge does not compromise an intact skin barrier. Perform intermediate level disinfection of these cups before use on another patient.

Here is an intermediate level disinfection protocol for cups that have not been exposed to blood or OPIM:

* Wear rubber utility gloves.

* Rinse used cups in water without splashing.

* Scrub cups with detergent.

* Inundate with EPA registered tuberculocidal germicide solution, or use a 1:10 - 1:100 solution of household bleach made fresh daily. (See Ch.13) Let them soak. Follow manufacturer's instructions on the germicidal solution.

* Drain cups into a sink, and allow to air dry.

Avoid or minimize blood removal by cupping. There are many alternative ways of moving stagnant blood, including moxibustion, herbs, compresses, acupressure, coining and Qi Gong exercises.

Risk Control Strategies:
Glove both hands for all cupping procedures.

Adjust cup pressure to avoid harm to skin at the cup's edges.

If a site is to be needled and cupped in the same treatment, cup first and needle second, to avoid blood contamination of cups.

Provide continuous hand support to cups that are drawing blood.

Position pump-induced vacuum cups to avoid blood entry into the valve area.

If cupping a site just previously needled, have paper toweling ready to absorb the blood. Use cups that are at least 40mm diameter at the base (2-3 ounce capacity).

Do not draw more than a teaspoon (~5ml) of blood into a cup.

Break the seal between the cup and skin gently, in an area on the rim where there is no blood or where there is the least likelihood of blood leakage.

Dispose of cups exposed to blood or OPIM, after the blood has been carefully absorbed or emptied down a drain.

After each use, perform intermediate level disinfection of cups that have not been exposed to blood or OPIM.

Use alternate ways to move stagnant blood, other than cupping.

Regulatory Compliance

Risks:
Compliance with regulatory requirements.

Discussion:
First ascertain whether the use of cupping is within your legal scope of practice. Then assess and document your training in cupping, prior to including it in your clinical repertoire.

Cupping devices are FDA Class III. If you choose to use cupping devices for treatment, implement the Class III device caveats from Chapter 12.

Risk Control Strategies:
Use cupping only if within your scope, training and competency.

If you choose to use cupping devices for treatment, implement the Class III device caveats from Chapter 12.

BEST PRACTICES

CUPPING

Inform patients about cupping marks and provide educational handout materials.

Obtain signed written informed consent for cupping.

Glove both hands for all cupping procedures.

Use clear walled pump-induced vacuum cups.

Do not use fire-induced vacuum cups.

Cupping contraindications:
* *frail elderly*   * *chronic cortisone users*
* *bleeding disorders*   * *anti-coagulant meds*
* *over non-intact skin areas*

Adjust pressure to avoid harm to skin at the cup's edges.

Adjust pressure to avoid causing blisters.

If a site is to be needled and cupped in the same treatment, cup first and needle second, to avoid blood contamination of cups.

Provide continuous hand support for cups drawing blood.

Position pump-induced vacuum cups to avoid blood contamination in the valve area.

If cupping a site just previously needled, have paper toweling ready to absorb blood. Use cups that are at least 40mm diameter at the base (2-3 ounce capacity).

Do not draw more than a teaspoonful (~5ml) of blood into a cup.

Break the seal between the cup and skin gently, in an area on the cup's rim where there is no blood or where there is the least likelihood of blood leakage.

Dispose of cups exposed to blood or OPIM, after the contaminant has been carefully absorbed or emptied down a closely situated drain.

After each use, perform intermediate level disinfection of cups that have not been exposed to blood or OPIM.

Use alternate way to move stagnant blood, other than cupping.

If you choose to use cupping devices for treatment, implement Class III device caveats from Chapter 12.

CHAPTER 17

COINING

The technical aspect of Coining opens with technical notes, followed by a discussion of bloodborne pathogen risks. We mention coining's mis-attribution to abuse, and close with regulatory compliance.

Technical Notes

Risks:
Dermal damage; excessive bruising.

Discussion:
Coining, known in Chinese as *gua sha*, is a dermal friction technique. It is a traditional Oriental family medical care procedure. It is also used by many acupuncturists to move stagnant blood in the muscle meridians, and to release exterior conditions. The friction implements are commonly the edge of a coin, or the edge of a ceramic Chinese-style high-edged soup spoon. A lubricant is applied to the skin, and re-applied as necessary during the process. Common lubricants include aromatic petroleum jelly based Vicks Vapo-Rub®, paraffin based Tiger Balm®, vegetable oil based massage lotions, skin moisturizers, and glycerin solutions.

Where stagnant blood is present, coining leaves a dark red slightly rough area, which later takes on the colors of a bruise as it resolves over several days. This redness is from the breakage of superficial capillary blood vessels, so in essence shallow bruising results.

Where no stagnant blood is present, the friction causes the skin to flush pink for an hour or less.

Coining is contraindicated over scars, raised moles, pimples, boils, and areas with broken skin or rashes. It is contraindicated on patients with bleeding disorders, and for those on anti-coagulant medications. The frail elderly who bruise with little provocation are not candidates for coining. Friction pressure must be adjusted to compensate for more fragile skin and/or fragile bones. These conditions are often encountered in the elderly, but may also be seen in younger persons as a result of extended cortisone use.

Coining should be managed so that its marks do not embarrass the patient. Inquire about upcoming events such as swim meets or social functions where a low cut dress might reveal coining marks. Schedule around these events. If coining on the back of the neck, advise the patient to wear a turtleneck shirt for several days.

Risk Control Strategies:
Do not perform coining over scars, raised moles, pimples, boils, and areas with broken skin or rashes.

Coining is contraindicated on the frail elderly, on patients with bleeding disorders, and on patients taking anti-coagulant medications.

Adjust friction pressure to compensate for more fragile skin and/or fragile bones.

Manage coining so that its marks do not embarrass the patient.

Bloodborne Pathogens

Risks:
Bloodborne pathogen exposures.

Discussion:
The coining lubricant sometimes turns a slightly pink color during the friction procedure. This color is from red blood cells which have been extravasated by pressure. Given that minute blood exposures can transmit viruses such as HBV and HIV, there is ample risk of disease transmission.

Latex exam gloves are a necessary PPE barrier for coining. <u>Never do coining without first gloving both hands</u>. Remain gloved until after clean up is completed.

If another procedure will be done on the same body area during this visit, do the other procedure first, and then do coining. If you must coin first, upon completion of coining clean up, remove your gloves and wash hands. Then don fresh gloves before returning to do other techniques requiring hand contact in the coined area. This work practice protects against contact with any minute quantity of blood remaining on the surface of the skin.

Petroleum jelly, paraffin, and vegetable oil based lubricants degrade latex gloves, making the gloves porous and prone to tear. Glycerin solutions are preferable in this regard, but are absorbed by the skin and need to be frequently re-applied.

To make a glycerin coining (or acupressure massage) lubricant, combine glycerin and water in the ratio of **8:1**, and mix well. If you prefer a thinner lubricant, increase the proportion of water. When mixing more of the solution than is immediately used, store the excess in labeled container. When mixing just as much as needed, a ~2 ounce clear plastic squeeze bottle can function as mixing container and dispenser.

Prior to beginning the coining procedure, dispense sufficient lubricant from the storage container into a ~2 ounce clear plastic squeeze bottle. Use the 2 ounce container as the dispenser during treatment. After treatment, dispose of any leftover lubricant, and then perform intermediate level decontamination of the 2 ounce dispenser. (See Ch. 13.) This protocol limits contamination to the small dispenser, and protects the larger container from becoming contaminated.

The friction implement should be clean, single use and disposable. While ceramic Chinese-style soup spoons could meet this criteria, they are also relatively expensive as single use disposable items. A 43mm diameter metal jar lid serves well as a friction device. These are obtainable by the gross from bottle companies at several cents per lid. A sample is shown in *Figure 17.1.* The lids must have a smooth rolled edge. This single use disposable device eliminates the risk of patient-to-patient disease transmission from re-used friction implements.

A modified technique is required to do coining with a jar lid. The lid is gripped with the distal joint of the thumb on top of the lid, and the flexed distal joint of the index finger under the lid. The grip is illustrated in *Figure 17.2.* A low angle of incidence is generally used, placing the lid's edge as flat to the skin as possible. As the lid's edge glides over the skin, so will the (gloved) index finger, which is positioned partially flexed under the lid's center.

A higher angle of incidence is used when working close to the lateral borders of the spine, along with a slight twist of the lid lateral to the direction of scraping.

Ch.17 Coining 201

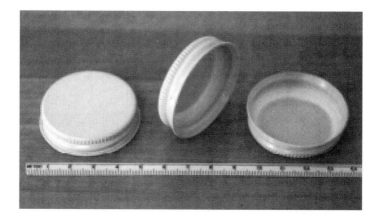

Figure 17.1 - Metal Jar Lid Friction Device

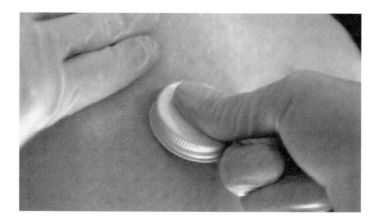

Figure 17.2 - Friction Lid In Use

Use a moist paper towel followed by a dry paper towel to clean the area of the body that has been coined. Discard excess lubricant and rinse the 2 ounce lubricant container. Then place it in a labeled holder for contaminated equipment awaiting decontamination. Now remove and dispose of gloves and wash hands. Dispose of used coining jar lids and gloves as contaminated waste.

Risk Control Strategies:
Glove both hands prior to coining and remain gloved until coining clean up is completed.

If another procedure will be done in the same body area during this visit, do the other procedure first, and then do coining. If you must coin first, then at the completion of coining cleanup, remove gloves, wash hands, and don new gloves for all other techniques requiring hand contact in the coined area.

Use a glycerin solution as a coining lubricant. Do not use petroleum or oil based lubricants, as they degrade latex gloves.

Use single- use disposable friction devices, such as metal jar lids (43mm diameter, smooth rolled edge).

Employ a small lubricant dispenser and fill it with enough lubricant for one treatment. After the procedure, dispose of the excess lubricant and perform an intermediate level decontamination of the small dispenser.

Mis-Attribution

Risks:
Mis-attribution of coining bruises to abuse.

Discussion:
Fresh coining can marks appear dreadful to individuals not familiar with them. Upon seeing swaths of reddened skin down the back of a child, caregivers have been known to contact child protective service agencies to investigate for abuse. Spouses of adult patients may react protectively as well, perceiving harm where the acupuncturist perceives help.

First educate your patient about coining, and then communicate the need for their outreach to educate family members and caregivers. Provide copies of an informative brochure to support this process.

Risk Control Strategies:
Educate patients and inform them of the need for their educational outreach to family members and other caregivers.

Provide educational handout materials.

Obtain signed written informed consent for coining.

Regulatory Compliance

Risks:
Compliance with regulatory requirements.

Discussion:
First ascertain whether the use of coining is within your legal scope of practice. Then assess and document your training in coining, prior to including it in your clinical repertoire.

Coining friction implements are arguably FDA Class III when intentionally sold (or used) as coining devices. (Ceramic soup spoons and metal jar lids are not intrinsically FDA regulated medical devices.) If you choose to use coining devices for treatment, heed the Class III device caveats from Chapter 12.

Risk Control Strategies:
Use coining only if within your scope, training and competency.

If you choose to use coining devices for treatment, implement the Class III device caveats from Chapter 12.

BEST PRACTICES

COINING

Coining is contraindicated:
*   *on scars*   *   *on raised moles*
*   *on pimples & boils*   *   *on non-intact skin*
*   *frail elderly*   *   *bleeding disorders*
*   *taking anti-coagulant medications*

Adjust friction pressure to compensate for more fragile skin and/or fragile bones.

Manage coining so that marks do not embarrass patient.

Glove both hands prior to coining and remain gloved until clean up is completed.

If another procedure will be done in the same body area during this visit, do the other procedure first, and then do coining. If you must coin first, at completion of the post-coining clean up, remove gloves and wash hands. Then don new gloves for all other techniques requiring hand contact in the coined area.

Use a glycerin solution as a coining lubricant. Do not use petroleum or oil based lubricants, as they degrade latex gloves.

Employ a small lubricant dispenser and fill with enough lubricant for one treatment. After the procedure, dispose of the excess lubricant and perform intermediate level decontamination of the small dispenser.

Use single-use disposable friction devices, such as metal jar lids (43mm diameter, smooth rolled edge).

Educate patients and inform them of the need for their educational outreach to family members and caregivers.

Provide educational handout materials.

Obtain signed written informed consent for coining.

If you choose to use coining devices for treatment, implement the Class III device caveats from Chapter 12.

CHAPTER 18

HERBS & SUPPLEMENTS

The technical aspect of Herbs & Supplements opens with discussion of labeling and medical claims, and then moves to a presentation of types and instances of adulteration. An abbreviated review of other potentially injurious herbs and supplements precedes consideration of risks associated with the herbal pharmacy. The chapter closes with a look at adverse events.

Labeling

Risks:
FDA regulatory compliance.

Discussion:
Herbal products and extracts (along with vitamins, etc.) are regulated as dietary supplements by the FDA under the Dietary Supplement Health & Education Act of 1994 (DSHEA). (See Chapter 12.)

The DSHEA requires that labels and printed materials accompanying dietary supplements make no medical claims. In the presence of medical claims, an herb is considered to be a drug, which invokes the context of drug regulations. In the absence of medical claims, an herb is a dietary supplement. Screen all herbal products for labeling compliance, and remove misbranded products. The FDA has detained many misbranded imported herbal preparations.

Make no medical claims for herbs that you prescribe. Explicitly disclaim medical intent: 'Herbal compounds are not intended to prevent, treat, mitigate or cure disease'. Communicate and chart only TOM indications for herbs (e.g. 'To nourish Liver Blood').

Refer to Herbal Compounding below for additional labeling issues.

Risk Control Strategies:
Assess your herbal products for DSHEA labeling compliance, and remove misbranded products.

Make no medical claims for herbs that you prescribe. Explicitly disclaim medical intent.

Communicate and chart only TOM energetic indications for herbs.

Assess your herbal products for compliance with your scope of practice regulations; remove non-compliant products.

Adulteration

Risks:
Illness or death from undeclared drugs, from toxic substances, or from heavy metals. FDA regulatory compliance. U.S. Fish & Wildlife Service compliance.

Discussion:
The FDA has identified a number of adulterated TOM herbal products. These may contain unsafe, undeclared, and/or regulated pharmaceutical components. A list is posted on the Internet at **http://www.fda.gov/ora/fiars/ora_import_ia6610.html**. Another list is provided on the California Society for Oriental

Medicine's website at **http://www.quickcom.net/csom/** Deaths and serious illnesses have resulted from ingestion of adulterated TOM patent medicines. (FDA 1991; CSOM 1997) Should any be present in your clinic, safely dispose of them.

Among Asian patent medicines listed by the above sources as containing undeclared pharmaceuticals are:

>   Chuifong Toukuwan   Hui Sheng Tsaitsaown
>
>   Chu Feng Shih Wan   Chui Fang Eng
>
>   Tung Shueh Pills   Jin Bu Huan Anodyne
>
>   Leung Pui Kee Cough Pills Bi Tong Pian
>
>   Bi Yan Pian   Ding Chuan Wan
>
>   Farfunpeiminkan Wan   Gan Mao Ling
>
>   Ma Hsing Zhi Ke Pian   Margarite Acne Pills
>
>   Pe Min Gan Wan   Yin Chiao
>
>   Zhong Gan Ling   Chong Ro Whan
>   Anti-Diarrheal

Asian patent medicines may also may contain ingredients considered toxic, particularly for children and during pregnancy. (CA Dept.Hlth.Svcs. 1992) While the TOM herbal tradition has used these substances with caution, modern biomedical and regulatory perspectives suggest even greater restraint. In light of the risks, substitute safer substances for all the toxic substances listed below:

    Aconite   Acorus   Borax

    Borneol   Bufonis   Buthus

    Cinnabar   Litharge   Minium

    Realgar   Semen Strychni

Never use Cinnabar, Litharge or Minium, as their heavy metals content accumulates in the body. Lead and cadmium have been detected in Asian herbal pills. (FDA 1991) Arsenic and/or mercury contamination have also been detected in Asian herbal ball preparations (Espinoza et al 1995), including:

    An Gong Niu Huang Wan   Da Huo Luo Wan

    Niu Huang Chiang Ya Wan   Niu Huang Ching Hsin Wan

    Ta Huo Lo Wan   Tsai Tsao Wan

    Dendrobium Moniliforme Night Sight Pills

Finally, U.S. Fish & Wildlife Service has confiscated Asian medicinal agents for alleged violations of the Endangered Species Act, Marine Mammal Act, and the global 1975 Convention on International Trade in Endangered Species of Wild Fauna & Flora (CITES). Listed animal species include Saiga Antelope, Bear, Leopard, Musk Deer, Pangolin, Rhino, Seal and Tiger. Wild

American ginseng is protected, and wild Chinese ginseng is considered endangered. (F&WS 1996)

Acupuncturists using imported Asian patents herbal compounds are advised to regularly consult resources for information on the presence of undeclared pharmaceuticals, toxic compounds, heavy metals contamination, and endangered species parts. (See Resources.) Review LD_{50} (lethal dose 50% of the time) data for TOM materia medica, and avoid substances possessing a small range between therapeutic and lethal doses.

In addition to acutely toxic substances, a number of herbs are considered potentially injurious. Refer to Potentially Injurious Herbs & Substances, below.

Risk Control Strategies:
Assess your herbal products for suspected adulteration with undeclared pharmaceuticals, toxic compounds, heavy metals contamination, or endangered species parts. If any are present, safely dispose of them.

Regularly consult resources for information on the presence of undeclared pharmaceuticals, toxic compounds, heavy metals contamination, and endangered species parts.

Review LD_{50} data for TOM materia medica, and avoid substances possessing a small range between therapeutic and lethal doses.

Other Potentially Injurious Herbs & Supplements

Risks:
Illness ascribed to herbs; state and federal regulatory compliance.

Discussion:
A number of herbs and supplements present known or suspected health risks. A few brief examples are provided.

Chaparral (Larrea tridentata) has been linked with liver disease, and has been voluntarily removed from the market. (Gordon 1995)

Comfrey is a suspected carcinogen. (Winship 1991; Couet et al 1996)

Ephedra (as extracted from Ma Huang) has a well documented abuse and injury potential, with over 500 reported adverse events in a two year period. (MMWR 1996) While the FDA is developing a regulatory policy, several states including OH, NY, FL and TX have already enacted controls. (FDA 1997a; Marandino 1997)

Germanium, on prolonged ingestion, has been linked to over 30 cases of nephrotoxicity, leading to death in some cases. (Tao & Bolger 1997)

L-tryptophan was implicated in over 1500 cases of Eosinophilia Myalgia Syndrome, and over 30 deaths resulted. The FDA suspects most - but not all- of the cases were related to impurities accidentally introduced by one manufacturer. (FDA 1996)

Vitamin A taken during pregnancy has been associated with injurious effects on the fetus. (Olson 1996; Polifka et al 1996)

It is an error to presume that over-the-counter natural herbs and dietary supplements are intrinsically safe. Use herbs and supplements based on demonstrable education, and stay current with the biomedical literature. Pay close attention to evolving state and federal regulatory actions.

Risk Control Strategies:
Remain well appraised of risks associated with herbs and supplements you prescribe. Use herbs and supplements within your legal scope of practice, based on demonstrable training.

Monitor state and federal regulatory actions.

Herbal Compounding

Risks:
Mis-identified herbs; impurities; non-standardized bio-activity; inadequate patient instruction.

Discussion:
Compounding is putting supplement ingredients together for a particular patient, as one might gather and package ingredients for an herbal tea. Compounding is not regulated by the FDA, beyond requirements of the DSHEA, but may be subject to state or local licensing requirements (i.e. repackaging license).

The transition of the TOM herbal pharmacy to America raises questions of the identity and quality of herbal substances, and issues of correct use by patients.

Herbalism relies on the correct identity and quality of herbs, and yet these are rarely tested. Practitioners presume that bulk herbs are what they are labeled to be. This is not always the case. Recently, packages labeled as plantain actually contained foxglove (a natural source of digitalis). The mislabeled foxglove was included in several commercial herbal preparations, with predictably dire consequences. (FDA 1997b) Closely inspect bulk herb stocks and arriving orders to determine accurate identity. Because more than one herbal substance may be present in bulk containers, inspect for inter-mixing. These tasks require a high level of botanical training.

The quality of herbs is also at issue. Are they clean and free of foreign matter? Do they contain pesticide or heavy metal residues? Are their bio-active constituents present in standard, greater or lesser amounts? Herbal pharmacies do not have the resources to biochemically assay their stocks. Large importers are more capable of assaying their products and supplying purity and bio-activity reports with each order. Encourage acupuncture organizations to meet with bulk herb importers to develop standards for testing and reporting.

Will herbal compounds be prepared and used as advised? When supplying one or more herbs to a patient, label the package and enclose written instructions. Indicate for whom it is intended, how it should be prepared, the serving size, when and for how long it should be taken, and any contraindications or precautions. List all ingredients in order from greatest to least. Include your name and telephone number, and the date the compound was supplied. You might also include an expiration date. Labeling software will simplify this task. Impeccable professional communication benefits patients and providers.

Risk Control Strategies:
Inspect all current and entering bulk herbs to determine accurate identity and lack of inter-mixing.

Encourage acupuncture organizations to meet with bulk herb importers to develop standards for herbal purity and bio-activity testing and reporting.

Label herbal compounds with: date; provider name and phone number; patient name; ingredients; instructions for preparation, serving size, timing and duration; precautions; and expiration date.

Adverse Events

Risks:
Side effects; allergic reactions; herb/drug interactions; prescriptive errors; accidental ingestion; product tampering.

Discussion:
When providing herbs, recall that it is not possible to biochemically alter complex living systems in one direction and one direction only. The strategy of polypharmacy is to minimize side effects of one substance by inclusion of other balancing substances. Nevertheless, side effects remains a distinct possibility. Patients have been hospitalized with gastritis caused by TOM herbs. (Anon 1996) Allergic reactions are another possibility. (See Chapter 9.) Initiating herbal treatment with a very small serving may help to reveal such adverse responses while incurring less harm. Be alert to the possibility of side effects, elicit patient reports of problems, and promptly respond with alteration or cessation of the herbs. Notify manufacturer and/or FDA at once.

Injurious interactions may occur between herbs and the pharmaceutical drugs that patients are taking concurrently. This territory has not been extensively researched. To minimize risk, review the physiologic effects of the biochemical constituents of each herb in a TOM formula, and then comparatively review the biochemistry of the patient's drugs. (Bensky et al 1986; Chen 1997; DFC 1998) Communication with the patient's biomedical providers may elicit pertinent drug biochemistry concerns.

Prescriptive errors can lead to adverse outcomes. Errors may be related not only to the quantity of herbs prescribed, but to the suitability of the herbs for the patient's condition. The necessity for accurate diagnosis is reflected in the highly developed state of diagnostic reasoning in TOM herbalism. Excellent training is the finest risk control.

The perfect herbal formula is only perfect for a given person at a given time, following clear instructions on preparation and use. Accidental ingestion by another person, particularly by a child, can lead to harm. Label herbal compounds as per recommendations given above. Select child resistant containers for herbal pills.

Product tampering remains a possibility. Select tamper resistant and tamper evident packaging for herbal and dietary supplements.

Risk Control Strategies:
Initiate herbal treatment with a small serving to reveal possible side effects or allergic responses.

Be alert to the possibility of side effects, elicit patient reports of problems, and promptly respond with alteration or cessation of herbs. Notify the manufacturer or FDA of problems at once.

Regularly review herbal adverse event literature.

To reduce risk of injurious herb/drug interactions, review the physiologic effects of the constituents of each herb in a TOM formula, and then comparatively review the biochemistry of the patient's drugs.

Select child resistant, tamper resistant and tamper evident packaging for herbal and dietary supplements.

BEST PRACTICES

HERBS & SUPPLEMENTS

Make no medical claims for herbs that you prescribe. Explicitly disclaim medical intent.

Communicate and chart only TOM indications for herbs.

Monitor state & federal herbal product regulatory actions.

Assess your herbal products for compliance with your scope of practice regulations; remove non-compliant products.

Assess your herbal products for DSHEA labeling compliance; remove mis-labeled products.

Assess your herbal products for suspected adulteration with undeclared pharmaceuticals, toxic compounds, heavy metals, or endangered species parts. If any are present, safely dispose of them.

Regularly consult resources for information on the presence of undeclared pharmaceuticals, toxic compounds, heavy metals, and endangered species parts.

Review LD_{50} data for TOM materia medica, and avoid substances possessing a small range between therapeutic and lethal doses.

Inspect all current and entering bulk herbs to determine accurate identity and lack of inter-mixing.

Encourage acupuncture organizations and bulk herb importers to jointly develop standards for herbal purity, bio-activity testing and reporting.

Label herbal compounds with: date; provider name and phone number; patient name; ingredients; instructions for preparation, serving size, timing and duration; precautions; and expiration date.

Select child resistant, tamper resistant and tamper evident packaging for herbal and dietary supplements.

Be alert to the possibility of side effects, elicit patient reports of problems, and promptly respond with alteration or cessation of herbs. Notify manufacturer or FDA of problems. Regularly review herbal adverse event literature.

To reduce risk of injurious herb/drug interactions, review physiologic effects of herbal constituents in the TOM formula, and compare with biochemistry of patient's drugs.

CHAPTER 19

ACUPRESSURE

In the technical aspect of Acupressure, we devise work practices and PPE protocols to control bloodborne pathogen risks. The chapter progresses to topics of excessive pressure application; sexual or improper touch; and regulatory compliance.

Bloodborne Pathogens

Risks:
Disease transmission from contact with blood and OPIM.

Discussion:
The risk of bloodborne pathogen transmission in acupressure can be controlled through work practices and PPE. These are applied to hand protection, treatment table sanitation, and acupressure device protocols.

Avoid unprotected hand contact with mucous membranes, cuts, pimples, boils or any other skin lesions on patients. HIV and HBV are not the only infective risks. For instance, *herpes zoster* is a transmissible virus present in the fresh lesions of shingles. If hand contact with non-intact skin, mucous membranes, blood or OPIM is likely or necessary, wear exam gloves as PPE on both hands. After treatment, remove and dispose of gloves as contaminated waste, and wash hands. Do not treat patients if your own hands are actively bleeding or exuding fluids (as from a weeping cut or rash).

Because petroleum and vegetable oil based massage lotions degrade latex, use a glycerin solution as an acupressure lotion when gloves are required. (See Chapter 17, Coining.) Afterwards, perform an intermediate level decontamination of the lubricant container. (See Ch. 13, Hygienic & Safety Practices)

The treatment table may become contaminated with blood and OPIM. To prevent this, provide a fresh treatment table cover and draping material for each patient. Perform an intermediate level decontamination of the table whenever it becomes contaminated, and at the end of every shift. Perform at least a low level decontamination before and after high risk patients. (See Ch. 13, Hygienic & Safety Practices, and Ch. 6, Universal Precautions)

Perform an intermediate level decontamination of acupressure devices after each use, if they have only contacted intact skin. If an acupressure device contacts non-intact skin, mucous membranes, blood or OPIM, it is a semi-critical instrument. It would require high level disinfection with a chemical sterilant (or autoclaving) prior to re-use. The preferable option is to dispose of the contaminated device.

Pointed acupressure devices (e.g. needle tipped probes), intended or likely to pierce the skin, are critical instruments. Sterilize prior to use, and dispose directly into a sharps container after use. This is in keeping with the principle that all critical and semi-critical instruments should be single use disposables. (See Ch.13, Equipment Sterilization & Disinfection.)

Risk Control Strategies:
Provide fresh treatment table cover and draping for each patient.

Do not treat patients if your hands are actively bleeding or exuding fluids.

Glove both hands for acupressure techniques involving contact with mucous membranes, non-intact skin areas, blood or OPIM. After treatment, remove and dispose of gloves as contaminated waste, and wash hands.

When doing acupressure wearing latex gloves, use a glycerin solution as a massage lotion in place of petroleum-based or oil-based products. Perform intermediate level decontamination of the lubricant container afterwards.

Perform intermediate level decontamination of the treatment table whenever it becomes contaminated, and at the end of every shift.

Perform at least a low level decontamination of the treatment table before and after high risk patients.

Perform intermediate level decontamination of acupressure devices after use on intact skin.

If an acupressure device contacts non-intact skin, mucous membranes, blood or OPIM, dispose of the device after use.

If an acupressure device is pointed, and intended or likely to pierce the skin (e.g. needle tipped probe), sterilize it prior to use, and dispose directly into a sharps container after use.

Excessive Pressure

Risks:
Excessive pressure causing tissue damage.

Discussion:

Yang styles of acupressure are characterized by the use of greater pressure and more vigorous manipulations. These styles are somewhat more prone to cause tissue damage, particularly in frail or osteoporotic patients. <u>Strong techniques</u> can be a point of practitioner pride. It is, however, a misplaced pride which would be better directed toward <u>appropriate techniques</u>.

Risk Control Strategies:

Adjust pressure and manipulation to the conditions of each body.

Sexual Or Improper Touch

Risks:

Sexual or improper touch (or touch that is perceived as such).

Discussion:

Acupressure at times presents several aspects of intimacy - a pair in privacy, semi-nudity, and with extensive touch. Either party (or both) may project an intimate relationship onto the therapeutic relationship. Sexual touch is not permissible, even if invited.

If an acupressure technique can potentially be interpreted as improper, explain the proposed technique in detail and proceed only with consent. Explain again while doing the technique, to further prevent mis-interpretation. Provide adequate draping to preserve modesty. Have a chaperone present during any treatment with a significant potential of being interpreted as improper. Let patients know that they are welcome to bring a chaperone.

As previously noted, whenever working on the lower pelvic area of a patient (regardless of gender), put on latex exam gloves first. In addition to the hygienic benefits, the PPE glove barrier psychologically reinforces the perception of the activity as clinical, for both patient and provider. (See Chapter 10, Sexual Boundaries)

Risk Control Strategies:
Provide adequate draping for patients.

Do not engage in sexual touch, even if invited.

If a technique has the potential of being interpreted as improper, explain in detail and proceed only with consent. Explain again while doing the technique.

Have a chaperone present during any treatment with significant potential of being interpreted as improper.

Whenever working on the lower pelvic area of a patient (regardless of gender), put on latex exam gloves first.

Regulatory Compliance

Risks:
Compliance with regulatory requirements.

Discussion:
First ascertain whether acupressure is within your legal scope of practice. Also determinewhether the acupressure devices you use are recognized as being within your scope of practice. Then assess and document your training, prior to including acupressure in your clinical repertoire.

Acupressure devices are FDA Class III. If you choose to use acupressure devices for treatment, implement the Class III device caveats from Chapter 12.

Risk Control Strategies:
Use acupressure and acupressure devices only if within your scope, training and competency.

If you choose to use acupressure devices for treatment, implement the Class III device caveats from Chapter 12.

BEST PRACTICES

ACUPRESSURE

Provide fresh treatment table cover and draping material for each patient.

Do not treat patients if your hands are actively bleeding or exuding fluids.

Glove both hands for acupressure techniques involving contact with mucous membranes, non-intact skin areas, blood or OPIM. After treatment, remove and dispose of gloves as contaminated waste, then wash hands.

When doing acupressure wearing latex gloves, use a glycerin solution as a massage lotion in place of oil based products. Perform intermediate level decontamination of the lubricant container afterwards.

Perform intermediate level decontamination of the treatment table whenever it becomes contaminated, and at the end of every shift.

Perform at least low level decontamination of the treatment table before and after high risk patients.

Perform intermediate level decontamination of acupressure devices after use on intact skin.

If an acupressure device contacts non-intact skin, mucous membranes, blood or OPIM, dispose of it after use.

If an acupressure device is pointed, and intended or likely to pierce the skin (e.g. needle tipped probe), sterilize it prior to use, and dispose directly into sharps container after use.

Adjust pressure and manipulation to the particular conditions of each body.

If a technique has the potential of being interpreted as improper, explain in detail and proceed only with consent. Explain again while doing the technique.

Have a chaperone present during any treatment with significant potential of being interpreted as improper.

Whenever working on the lower pelvic area of a patient (regardless of gender), put on latex exam gloves first.

If you choose to use acupressure devices for treatment, implement the Class III device caveats from Chapter 12.

CHAPTER 20

ELECTROACUPUNCTURE

The technical aspect of Electroacupuncture opens with technical notes, describing a variety of devices and listing contraindications. The chapter closes with regulatory compliance issues.

Technical Notes

Risks:
Contraindicated uses and hazards.

Discussion:
Electroacupuncture is a general term encompassing electro-diagnosis, electronic point location, and electro-stimulation techniques. Electro-diagnosis involves the interpretation of conductivity or resistance measurements at acupuncture points. A small reference current is applied to determine acupoint response. Several systems of electro-diagnosis have evolved, including Vegatest, EAV (Voll), Auriculotherapy (Nogier), and Ryodo-raku (Nakatani). Electronic point locators are similar but simpler devices which respond to decreases in skin resistance with audible or visible signals instead of electronic gauge readings.

Electro-stimulation devices supply direct current in a variety of wave forms, frequencies, patterns and current strengths. Standard acupuncture electro-stimulation devices are capable of supplying up to ~60mA current to inserted needles. Electrical muscle stimulators (EMS) produce a similar current. Transcutaneous electronic nerve stimulators (TENS) supply a maximum of ~80mA via surface electrodes. Microcurrent TENS devices deliver only 200-900uA. (1000uA = 1mA)

The safest practice is to use the lowest current necessary. Excessive current can cause electrical burns, and could induce cardiac arrhythmias or seizures. Painful levels of current are excessive.

Electro-stimulation units are predominantly battery powered. Line current devices should be Underwriters Laboratory (UL) listed and have a ground wire (three-prong) plug, connected to a wall socket with a ground fault circuit interrupter (GFCI). To minimize accidental shock hazards, avoid line current devices.

The primary medical contraindication for electro-diagnosis relates to inappropriate use in place of other diagnostic techniques. Exercise particular caution in forming, charting, and verbalizing biomedical diagnostic conclusions based on electro-diagnosis, in the absence of confirming biomedical diagnostic tests. Exclusive reliance on electro-diagnosis engenders risks of patient harm related to erroneous and missed biomedical and TOM diagnoses.

There are no apparent medical contraindications for point locators.

Electro-stimulation devices are contraindicated for certain patients and placements (Naeser & Wei 1994; NAF 1997; OMS 1996):

* seizure disorder * cardiac pacemaker
* cardiac disease * electronic implants
* malignancy * pregnancy
* pain of undetermined etiology
* patients with ECG monitors & alarms
* over carotid sinuses * transcerebrally

*	transthoracically	*	near heart
*	near eyes	*	on non-intact skin

Silver needles readily electrolyze when used as electrodes. This increases risk of breakage and also may disperse toxic levels of silver into tissues. Do not use silver needles for electro-acupuncture. (NAF 1997)

Electrode wires clipped to inserted acupuncture needles can pull on those needles. A needle might be pulled out, or pulled down deeper into the body than is safe. Address this problem by stabilizing the wires in a way that reduces drag on the needles. An effective technique is to tape the wires to the patient.

Risk Control Strategies:
Avoid contraindicated uses and placements.

Use battery powered devices and the lowest current necessary.

Do not use silver needles for electro-stimulation.

Tape electrode wires to reduce needle drag.

Regulatory Compliance

Risks:
Compliance with scope of practice and FDA regulations.

Discussion:
At least 11 states explicitly include electroacupuncture in statutory definitions of scope of practice. (CAAOM 1997) Regulations in

other states accommodate certain electroacupuncture practices. It is important to determine whether electro-diagnosis, electronic point location, and/or electro-stimulation are within your scope. Select devices whose capabilities do not exceed your scope. Several devices perform location, diagnostic measurement and stimulation. Assess and document your training for those aspects within your scope, prior to initiating clinical use.

Standard electroacupuncture devices are FDA Class III, limited to investigational use. Substitute Class II devices when possible, as approved by your state regulatory board and professional association.

Many TENS and EMS models are Class II devices, cleared for marketing to qualified practitioners, and for sale to patients on prescription of a qualified practitioner. Labeled uses of TENS devices are for chronic intractable pain and post-surgical traumatic acute pain. Labeled uses of EMS devices are muscle spasm relaxation; prevention or retardation of disuse atrophy; muscle reeducation; maintain or increase range of motion; increase local blood circulation; prevent thrombosis in bedridden patients. All other indications are off-label, and may not be advertised. Make no claims of safety or efficacy for off-label uses, and do not advertise off-label uses.

Additionally there are Class II galvanic skin response (GSR) and skin potential measurement devices, which might be substituted for Class III electro-diagnostic devices (although the substitutes lack electro-stimulation treatment capabilities).

For investigational use of electroacupuncture devices, follow all FDA requirements for research.

Ch.20 Electroacupuncture

If you choose to use Class III electroacupuncture devices for treatment, implement these caveats (and refer to Ch.12):

Do not advertise use of Class III devices. It is illegal to advertise the brand names of Class III devices you use (e.g. 'EAV Dermatron' or 'Vegatest'). Do not sell Class III devices to patients, nor provide such devices for home use.

Document supportive evidence for your uses of electroacupuncture.

Inform patients that the device and its indications are not FDA cleared, using signed written consent. Explicitly state that no medical claims of safety or efficacy are made for the device.

Provide electroacupuncture in addition to biomedical and TOM standards of care. For instance, confirm electro-diagnostic findings with referral for standard biomedical tests, rather than foregoing referral for biomedical tests.

Couch any electro-diagnostic conclusions provisionally, within the context of TOM, and with suitable disclaimers. For instance: 'These electric measurements suggest an energetic imbalance in the gall bladder, according to TOM theories. This could occur in the absence of any biomedical pathology in that organ. If you are experiencing gall bladder disease symptoms, you should consult your biomedical primary care provider for diagnosis. Biomedical diagnoses cannot be established on the basis of TOM electro-diagnosis.'

Risk Control Strategies:

Determine whether electro-diagnosis, electronic point location, and/or electro-stimulation are within your scope of practice.

Select devices whose capabilities do not exceed your scope.

Assess and document your training for those aspects within your scope, prior to initiating clinical use.

Substitute Class II for Class III devices when possible, as approved by your state regulatory board and professional association.

For investigational use of electroacupuncture devices, follow all FDA requirements for research.

If you choose to provide treatment use of Class III electro-acupuncture devices:
> Do not advertise use and do not sell or provide devices to patients.
> Document supportive evidence for your uses of electro-acupuncture.
> Inform patients in a written consent process that the devices and indications are not FDA cleared.
> Provide electroacupuncture in addition to biomedical and TOM standards of care.
> Exercise caution in forming, charting and verbalizing biomedical diagnostic conclusions based on electro-diagnosis.

BEST PRACTICES

ELECTROACUPUNCTURE

Determine if electro-diagnosis, electronic point location, and electro-stimulation are within your scope of practice.

Assess and document your training for those aspects within your scope, prior to initiating clinical use.

Select devices whose capabilities do not exceed your scope.

Substitute Class II for Class III devices when possible, as approved by your state regulatory board and professional association.

Use battery powered devices and lowest current necessary.

Do not use silver needles for electro-stimulation.

Tape electrode wires to reduce needle drag.

Avoid electro-stimulation in these patients and placements:
- *   *seizure disorder*   *   *cardiac pacemaker*
- *   *cardiac disease*   *   *electronic implants*
- *   *malignancy*   *   *pregnancy*
- *   *pain of undetermined etiology*
- *   *patients with ECG monitors & alarms*

* *over carotid sinuses* * *transcerebrally*
* *transthoracically* * *near heart*
* *near eyes* * *on non-intact skin*

For investigational use of electroacupuncture devices, follow all FDA requirements for research.

If you choose to provide treatment use of Class III electro-acupuncture devices:
> *Do not advertise use and do not sell or provide devices to patients.*
> *Document supportive evidence for your uses of electro-acupuncture.*
> *Inform patients in a written consent process that the devices and indications are not FDA cleared.*
> *Provide electroacupuncture in addition to biomedical and TOM standards of care.*
> *Exercise particular caution in forming, charting, and verbalizing biomedical diagnostic conclusions based on electro-diagnosis.*

CHAPTER 21

LASER DEVICES

In the technical aspect of Laser Devices, technical notes and hazard control sections address risks of lasers, and risk control responses. The chapter closes with a look at regulatory issues.

Technical Notes

Risks:
Laser hazards & contraindicated uses.

Discussion:
Laser is the acronym for Light Amplification by Stimulated Emission of Radiation. Laser light is very coherent and monochromatic, in marked contrast to common forms of light.

Lasers are classed by hazard levels based on radiant power output. The FDA defines four classes and several sub-classes, increasing in hazard from Class I to Class IV. Biostimulation lasers, also known as cold lasers, soft lasers, and low level laser therapy devices, are generally Class IIIa or Class IIIb. Class IIIa lasers produce 1 to 5mW, while Class IIIb outputs range from 5mW to 500mW (.005 - .5W). Each class of laser must carry a warning label prescribed by the FDA. (21CFR1040.10) FDA power output classifications are different than medical device classifications.

The most common serious injury from laser light is eye damage. Directly viewed laser light is condensed by the pupil, with up to a

100,000 fold increase in radiant power received at the retina. Permanent blindness can result. Class IIIa and IIIb lasers pose an acute intrabeam viewing hazard. Class IIIb lasers present diffuse ocular hazards, and skin burn hazards from direct radiation, when near the 500mW output limit. (OSHA 1995; Naeser & Wei 1994) In addition to direct, reflected and scattered radiation hazards, lasers may also present fire and electrical risks.

Class IV lasers have stringent hazard control measures associated with their use. They cut, cauterize and vaporize tissue, and have caused fatalities from accidental burns. Never use Class IV lasers as biostimulation laser devices.

Research into the biologic effects and therapeutic benefits of biostimulation lasers is still at an early stage. Contraindications include eye exposure; use on cancerous growths; use in pregnancy; and use over unclosed fontanelles in infants or small children. (Naeser & Wei 1994)

Calculations of output energy per second and energy density per cm^2 are necessary to determine safe and what may be regarded as therapeutic laser light exposure times. The fundamental formula is $\mathbf{J = W \times S}$, where J = energy in joules, W = power in watts, and S = time in seconds. Calculations are more complex for pulsed lasers.

Risk Control Strategies:
Avoid contraindicated uses:
- * on or near eyes
- * in pregnancy
- * on cancerous growths
- * over unclosed fontanelles

Calculate safe and therapeutically optimal exposure times.

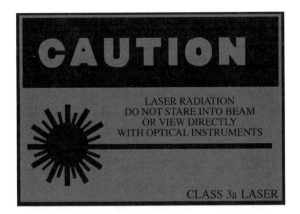

*Figure 21.1 - CAUTION Laser Use Area Sign
(yellow background, black symbol)*

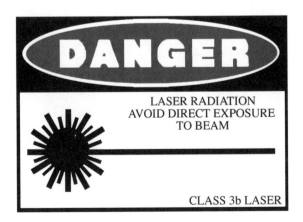

*Figure 21.2 - DANGER Laser Use Area Sign
(red symbol, red surrounding 'danger')*

Hazard Controls

Risks:
Thermal and photochemical damage to eyes and skin.

Discussion:
Hazard controls are recommended (but not yet mandated) by regulatory agencies. Mandated or not, safe operating practices are both prudent and ethical. American National Standards Institute (ANSI) has published relevant laser safety standards in ANSI Z136.1 and ANSI Z136.3. (ANSI 1993; ANSI 1996) Among FDA and ANSI laser safety standards, the following are emphasized.

Class IIIa lasers are not normally hazardous, except for direct eye exposure. It is prudent to post a CAUTION sign with the laser hazard symbol in the use area. Refer to ***Figure 21.1.*** The lasers must have the prescribed warning label, and are best stored in a locked drawer when not in use. Never directly view the beam.

Many Class IIIa laser pens used in acupuncture are identical in output to laser pointing devices used by speakers. Do not presume that they are therefore not hazardous. Two cases of eye injury from laser pointing devices were reported in 1996. (Rockwell 1996)

Hazard controls for Class IIIa lasers are far simpler than for Class IIIb lasers. Standards for Class IIIb laser hazard control include:

* DANGER sign with the laser hazard symbol, posted in the use area. Refer to ***Figure 21.2.***

* Devices must have the prescribed warning label.

* Store devices in a locked container when not in use.

* Laser eye protection glasses (matched to the type and output of the laser) worn by the patient. See Resources.

* Exclude spectators or other individuals from area during use.

* Curtain barriers defining nominal hazard zone, and preventing reflected and through-window exposures.

* Operator has demonstrable laser use and safety training.

* Device use limited to authorized personnel.

* Written standard operating procedures.

A statement of <u>standard operating procedures</u> for Class IIIb lasers might include:

* Calculate and confirm dosimetry as safe.

* Confirm laser informed consent document in patient records.

* Avoid exposure to eyes; on cancerous growths; in pregnancy; and over unclosed fontanelles in infants or small children.

* Clear extraneous personnel from area.

* Close barrier curtains, minimize reflected light hazards.

* Position patient safely to minimize potential eye exposure.

* Provide patient with PPE (laser safety eyewear).

* Set timer for exposure duration.

* Place laser aperture on acupuncture point and stabilize.

* Start laser emission.

* Stop emission before lifting laser aperture from acupuncture point.

* Lock laser device on completion of procedure.

* Chart each point and duration of treatment.

Always provide laser safety eyewear as PPE for the patient when using any laser device. Provide laser safety eyewear as PPE for the acupuncturist if using the most powerful Class IIIb devices. Consult Resources for laser safety eyewear sources.

Risk Control Strategies:
Implement ANSI Z136 safety standards for hazard class of laser device.

Never use Class IV laser devices.

Document safe operating procedures.

Always provide laser safety eyewear for the patient when using any laser device. Provide laser safety eyewear for the acupuncturist if using the most powerful Class IIIb devices.

Regulations & Standards

Risks:
Scope of practice compliance; FDA compliance; ANSI standards compliance.

Discussion:
Florida, Massachusetts, New Mexico and Washington identify laser therapy in statute as part of the scope of acupuncture practice. (CAAOM 1997) Other states may have regulatory provisions including lasers in the scope of acupuncture practice. Ascertain that lasers are within your scope of practice prior to initiating use.

Where it is within legal scope, competency is a prerequisite to use. Competency is based on training in laser safety and use protocols. (See Resources.)

The medical use of lasers is not yet fully regulated. However, regulatory concern with laser use is increasing. OSHA has not enacted worker safety standards other than for the construction industry. Most states with laser safety legislation have exempted medical providers. Review laser law in your state to determine its impact. ANSI has published guidelines for safety and use. Adherence to the ANSI standards is voluntary, but it is practically required from a liability perspective.

The FDA defines biostimulation lasers as Class III devices, cleared only for investigational use. When using lasers in an investigational protocol, follow all FDA rules for research. (See Chapter 12.) If research subjects are required to pay for devices or associated services, charges must be at no more than costs, as no profits may be made. Charges must be approved by the IRB. Subjects must be informed of charges in a written consent process.

If you choose to provide treatment use of biostimulation lasers, implement these caveats (and refer to Chapter.12):

Do not advertise use and do not sell or provide devices to patients.

Use laser devices in ways that do not pose significant hazards. Implement ANSI standards for laser safety.

Document supportive evidence for your uses of lasers.

Inform patients in a written consent process that the medical device and indications for the device are not FDA cleared. Explicitly state that no medical claims are made for the device.

Provide biostimulation laser therapy in addition to, not in lieu of, biomedical and TOM standards of care.

Risk Control Strategies:
Use laser devices only if within your legal scope of practice, and within your competency based on training.

For investigational use of biostimulation lasers, follow all FDA requirements for research.

If you choose to provide treatment use of biostimulation lasers:
> Do not advertise use and do not sell or provide devices to patients.
> Use laser devices in ways that do not pose significant hazards. Implement ANSI safety standards.
> Document supportive evidence for your uses of lasers.
> Inform patients in a written consent process that the device and indications are not FDA cleared.
> Provide biostimulation laser therapy in addition to, not in lieu of, biomedical and TOM standards of care.

BEST PRACTICES

LASER DEVICES

Use laser devices only if within your legal scope of practice and within your competency supported by training.

Review and comply with laser safety laws in your state.

Avoid contraindicated uses:
- ** on or near eyes*
- ** on cancerous growths*
- ** in pregnancy*
- ** over unclosed fontanelles in infants, children*

Calculate safe and estimated therapeutic exposure times for each laser device.

Implement ANSI Z136 safety standards for the hazard class of laser devices you use.

Never use Class IV lasers as biostimulation devices.

Document safe operating procedures.

Always provide laser safety eyewear for the patient.

Provide laser safety eyewear for the acupuncturist if using the most powerful Class IIIb devices.

For investigational use of lasers, follow all FDA research regulations.

If you choose to use biostimulation lasers clinically:
> *Do not advertise use, and do not sell or provide devices to patients.*
> *Use lasers in ways that are not hazardous. Comply with ANSI laser safety standards.*
> *Document supportive evidence for your uses of lasers.*
> *Inform patients in a written consent process that devices and indications are not FDA cleared.*
> *Provide laser therapy in addition to biomedical and TOM standards of care.*

CHAPTER 22

MAGNETIC DEVICES

The technical aspect of Magnetic Devices opens with technical notes and a list of contraindications. The regulatory compliance section addresses the use of magnets within scope of practice and Class III device regulations.

Technical Notes

Risks:
Contraindicated uses.

Discussion:
The ambient magnetic field strength at the Earth's surface is about .5 Gauss. The effects of placing 500 Gauss magnets on acupuncture points for varying periods of time have not been fully elucidated. Discussion continues on the merits of placing the negative as versus the positive field toward the body. If you decide to use magnets, use them conservatively with reference to their strength, number, duration and placements.

Contraindications include use on patients with cardiac pacemakers, defibrillators, electrical implants, or during pregnancy. Caution is advised in placing magnets around the head. (Total Health 1997; Becker 1990)

Certain individuals develop contact dermatitis from metals or adhesive tapes. Inquire on your new patient medical history form about skin irritation from contact with metals and adhesive tapes.

Risk Control Strategies:
Use magnets conservatively with respect to their strength, number, duration and placements.

Do not use magnets on patients with cardiac pacemakers, defibrillators, electrical implants, or during pregnancy. Caution is advised in placing magnets around the head.

Inquire on your new patient medical history form about skin irritation from contact with metals or adhesive tapes.

Regulatory Compliance

Risks:
Compliance with regulatory requirements.

Discussion:
First ascertain whether the use of magnetic devices is within your legal scope of practice. Then assess and document your training in the therapeutic use of magnets, prior to including this form of therapy in your clinical repertoire.

Magnets are FDA Class III devices when used for medical treatments, and are not cleared for marketing. The FDA has detained a number of consumer magnetic devices due to labeling that includes medical claims. Assess your clinic's stock of magnetic products for labeling compliance, and remove non-compliant products.

For investigational use of magnets, comply with all FDA research requirements. (See Chapter 12.)

If you choose to use magnets for treatment, outside of research contexts, implement Class III device caveats (See Chapter 12):

Let use be visible only to your patents. Do not advertise or sell magnets as medical devices. If magnets are not labeled, intended, used or held out to be medical devices, then their sale is not FDA regulated.

Document supportive evidence for your medical use of magnets.

Inform patients in a written consent process that magnets and indications for them are not FDA cleared as safe or effective. Explicitly state that no medical claims are made for the devices (e.g. 'Magnetic devices are not intended to diagnose, prevent or treat disease'). Thereafter, one might carefully express a TOM perspective on magnets as energetic influences on the body, without ever stating that they are therapeutically effective.

Provide magnet therapy in addition to, not in lieu of, TOM and biomedical standards of care.

Risk Control Strategies:
Use magnets only if within your scope, training and competency.

Assess your clinic's stock of magnetic products for labeling compliance, and remove non-compliant products.

Follow FDA research protocols for investigational use of magnets.

If you choose to provide treatment use of magnets:
- Do not advertise or sell magnets as medical devices.
- Document supportive evidence for your uses.
- Inform patients in a written consent process that magnets and their indications are not FDA cleared.
- Provide magnet therapy in addition to biomedical and TOM standards of care.

BEST PRACTICES

MAGNETIC DEVICES

Use magnets only if within your scope, training and competency.

Assess your clinic stock of magnetic devices for labeling compliance; remove non-compliant devices.

Use magnets conservatively with respect to their strength, number, duration and placements.

Contraindications for magnets:
- *cardiac pacemakers*
- *defibrillators*
- *electrical implants*
- *pregnancy*

Caution is advised in placing magnets around the head.

Inquire on new patient medical history form about skin irritation from contact with metals or adhesive tapes.

For investigational use of magnets, follow all FDA regulations.

If you choose to provide treatment use of magnets:
> *Do not advertise or sell magnets as medical devices.*
> *Document supportive evidence for your uses of magnets.*
> *Inform patients in a written consent process that magnets & indications are not FDA cleared.*
> *Provide magnet therapy in addition to biomedical and TOM standards of care.*

APPENDICES

A.		FORM & RECORD EXAMPLES	253
	1.	EMERGENCY ACTION PLAN EXAMPLE	253
	2.	FIRE PREVENTION PLAN EXAMPLE	256
	3.	MATERIAL SAFETY DATA SHEET EXAMPLE: ISOPROPYL ALCOHOL	258
	4.	HAZARD COMMUNICATION PROGRAM EXAMPLE	265
	5.	HBV VACCINE DECLINATION FORM	267
	6.	EMPLOYEE MEDICAL RECORD	268
	7.	EMPLOYEE MEDICAL RECORD RELEASE FORM	269
	8.	EXPOSURE INCIDENT REPORT	270
	9.	HEALTHCARE PROFESSIONAL'S POST EXPOSURE WRITTEN OPINION	271
	10.	POST EXPOSURE EVALUATION RECORD	272

11. BLOODBORNE PATHOGENS EXPOSURE CONTROL PLAN EXAMPLE   273

B. HAZARD COMMUNICATION
    29 CFR 1910.1200   281

C. BLOODBORNE PATHOGENS STANDARD
    29 CFR 1910.1030   297

EMERGENCY ACTION PLAN EXAMPLE

Established For:_____
_____ (Name and Address of practice)

In compliance with 29 CFR 1910.38, 1910.157 and 1910.165, and in the interest of injury prevention, the management staff of this practice hereby defines an Emergency Action Plan. This written program will be located in: _____
_____, and is available for review by any interested employees. Additionally, copies will be given to all current and new employees.

Emergency Evacuation
In case of fire, toxic chemical release, or explosion in the building, we require a total and immediate evacuation of all employees with non-essential duties. An appended FLOOR PLAN MAP indicates emergency escape routes. Exit doors are located: _____.

Employees are instructed to use the nearest safe route, to move away from exit doors and away from the building, and to assemble at an exterior safe area so that they may be accounted for. The exterior safe area is located: _____
_____.

For an Alarm System compliant with 1910.165, smoke detectors are installed. and are regularly maintained and tested. When a smoke detector alarm sounds (other than in a test), the Acupuncturist will immediately attempt to verify the location and nature of the possible fire emergency. She will then announce directions to patients, employees, and other occupants, advising on whether the alarm is false, real or undetermined. Real and undetermined alarms require evacuation. Direct voice communication (shouting) will also be used to warn of fire and other emergencies.

Portable fire extinguishers are provided in the workplace, for use by designated employees. Acupuncturist and Receptionist have been designated for extinguisher use.

Employees With Essential Duties
In an emergency requiring evacuation, the following employees will delay their own evacuation, only when it is prudent to do so without risk of immediate personal harm, to complete essential duties, as follows:

A. Receptionist: will telephone 911 to summon emergency aid; will direct all waiting room occupants to nearest safe exit route, and will prevent their re-entry to the building while hazards remain and until emergency aid personnel assume this duty; and finally will assist Acupuncturist by directing patients to nearest safe exit route. As an employee designated to use portable fire extinguishers, she will use fire extinguishers when appropriate to control small fires, based on training provided by the employer.

B. Acupuncturist: will announce to all patients the nature of the emergency and the appropriate response required. Whenever it is the safer option, the Acupuncturist will remove all acupuncture needles from patients before evacuating patients and herself. In the absence of Receptionist, the Acupuncturist will assume Receptionist's essential duties. As an employee designated to use portable fire extinguishers, she will use fire extinguishers when appropriate to control small fires, based on training provided by the employer.

Accounting For Employees After Emergency Evacuation
Of employees assembling at the safe area after emergency evacuation, one will note the number of employees unaccounted for. The Acupuncturist is assigned responsibility for this task, but it must be assumed by another employee if the Acupuncturist is unaccounted for.

Rescue and Medical Aid Duties - Emergency Medical Plan
Employees are not to return to the premises after evacuation and while hazardous conditions persist. When rescue and emergency medical aid is required, emergency medical service providers will be summoned by dialing 911.

The Acupuncturist is designated as first responder for medical emergencies. Our facility first aid supplies are located: _____
_____. Monthly inspection, maintenance, decontamination, and re-supply whenever necessary of the first aid supplies is the responsibility of: _____ (Name, Job Title).

Means of Reporting Fires & Other Emergencies
The preferred means of reporting fires and other emergencies is by telephone, dialing 911, and advising the dispatcher about the nature of the emergency. If it is safe to do so, this may be done on the premises; otherwise an off-premises telephone should be used.

Plan Informational Contacts
For further information or explanation of duties under this plan, contact: _____(Name, Job Title)

Training
Before initial implementation of this plan, the employer will train every employee in safe and orderly emergency evacuation procedures, and in the employee's designated responsibilities or designated actions under the plan. Training will be repeated whenever the employee's duties change under this plan, and whenever the plan is changed. New employees will be trained prior to initial assignment.

Employees designated for fire extinguisher use will receive training upon initial assignment, covering: principles of fire extinguisher use; hazards of first stage fire fighting; hands-on experience using an extinguisher; and when to evacuate. Training will be repeated at least annually.

Employees designated as first responders will receive: bloodborne pathogens training, offer of HBV vaccination, appropriate PPE, and all other requirements under 29CFR1910.1030 Bloodborne Pathogens Standard.

Evaluation and Review

_____(Name, Job Title) is responsible for reviewing this Emergency Action Plan annually or as needed, and updating as needed.

Emergency Action Plan Adopted on this date:_____,
By_____ (highest mgmnt. official)

FIRE PREVENTION PLAN EXAMPLE

Established For:_____
_____ (Name and Address of practice)
In compliance with 29 CFR 1910.38, 1910.157 and 1910.165, and in the interest of injury prevention, the management staff of this practice hereby defines a Fire Prevention Plan. This written program will be located in: _____
_____, and is available for review by any interested employees. Additionally, copies will be given to all current and new employees.

Fire Hazards

    1. Isopropyl Alcohol Description: FLAMMABLE liquid. Vapors may travel to a source of ignition and flash back. CONTAINERS MAY EXPLODE IN FIRE. POISONOUS GASES ARE PRODUCED IN FIRE.

    Control Procedures: Store in cool ventilated area, in tightly capped upright containers. Store to avoid contact with STRONG OXIDIZERS (such as CHLORINE, BROMINE, and FLUORINE) since violent reactions occur. Label containers as FLAMMABLE. Do not handle near open flames or smoking. Handle in well ventilated areas. If Isopropyl Alcohol is spilled or leaked, take the following steps: Restrict persons not wearing protective equipment from area of spill or leak until cleanup is complete; Remove all ignition sources; Ventilate area of spill or leak; Absorb liquids in vermiculite, dry sand, earth, or a similar material and deposit in sealed containers; Keep Isopropyl Alcohol out of a confined space, such as a sewer, because of the possibility of an explosion, unless the sewer is designed to prevent the buildup of explosive concentrations.

    Fire Protection Equipment: Dry chemical, CO2, water spray, or alcohol foam extinguishers, for use by designated employees. For large spills and all fires, call 911.

    2. Moxibustion Description: Indirect moxibustion warming devices consist of: Infrared heat lamps. If heat lamp element contacts flammable material, fire could result. Direct moxibustion devices consist of butane lighters, incense sticks, and moxa wool cones. The lighter ignites an incense stick, which is used to ignite a small moxa wool cone secured to an acupuncture point. Incense stick and moxa wool burn as embers, and live embers are capable of igniting a fire.

    Control Procedures: Heat lamps are equipped with element guards to prevent contact with flammable material. Heat lamps are equipped with heavy bases to reduce risk of tipping over and contacting flammable material. Store lighters in cool area. Provide holder for incense stick while in use. Extinguish incense sticks immediately after use. Moxa wool cones are secured with a slip of petroleum jelly to prevent their accidental detachment. It is our policy to require that a cup of water be available at all times during direct moxibustion treatments, to quench embers, should the need arise. Smoke detectors will be located to minimize false alarms from the small amount of smoke produced in direct moxibustion.

Fire Protection Equipment: Water spray, dry chemical, or CO2, for use by designated employees. Direct moxibustion embers can be extinguished by compression, or with water. For all fires, call the Fire Department, 911.

3. Cupping Description: Pump-induced vacuum devices.

Control Procedures: It is our policy to not allow employees to use fire-induced vacuum cupping. All fire-induced vacuum cups have been replaced with pump-induced vacuum cups. Cupping is no longer a fire hazard.

Fire Protection Equipment: none required.

Fire Prevention Contact
Name & Job Title of person responsible for control of fire hazards:
_____.

Housekeeping Procedures
Flammable and combustible waste will be removed from the premises on the following schedule: At the end of every shift, and whenever waste containers are full.

Training
All current employees will be trained in fire hazards to which they are exposed. Each new employee will be trained prior to initial assignment. Employees designated for fire extinguisher use will receive training upon initial assignment, covering: principles of fire extinguisher use; hazards of first stage fire fighting; hands-on experience using an extinguisher; and when to evacuate. Training will be repeated at least annually.

Maintenance
All heating systems will receive maintenance checks at least annually. All infrared lamps will be inspected for safety and element guard attachment security at least quarterly.

Portable Fire Extinguishers
Portable fire extinguishers are intended for use by designated employees. Extinguishers will be inspected, maintained and tested as follows: Annual check by person trained to recognize problems; Recording of annual maintenance date on tag attached to extinguisher; Monthly visual check of charge; Hydrostatic testing either every 5 years for CO2 and wet chemical types, or 12 years for dry chemical and Halon types, performed by a fire extinguisher maintenance company.

Evaluation and Review
_____(Name, Job Title) is responsible for reviewing this Fire Prevention Plan annually or as needed, and updating as needed.
Fire Prevention Plan Adopted on this date:_____,
By_____ (highest mgmnt. official)

MATERIAL SAFETY DATA SHEET
ISOPROPYL ALCOHOL

Common Name: Isopropyl Alcohol   CAS Number: 67-63-0   DOT Number: UN 1219
Date: September, 1988

HAZARD SUMMARY
* Isopropyl Alcohol can affect you when breathed in and by passing through your skin.
* There is an increased risk of cancer associated with the manufacturing of Isopropyl Alcohol.
* Exposure can cause irritation of the eyes, nose, mouth, and throat.
* Overexposure may cause headaches, drowsiness, clumsiness, unconsciousness, and death.
* Contact may irritate the skin. Repeated skin exposure can cause itching, a rash, and drying and cracking.
* Isopropyl Alcohol is a FLAMMABLE LIQUID and a FIRE HAZARD.

IDENTIFICATION
Isopropyl Alcohol is a colorless liquid. Rubbing alcohol is a solution of Isopropyl Alcohol. It is used as a solvent and in making many commercial products.

REASON FOR CITATION
* Isopropyl Alcohol is on the Hazardous Substance List because it is regulated by OSHA and cited by ACGIH, DOT, NFPA and EPA.
* This chemical is on the Special Health Hazard Substance List because it is FLAMMABLE.
* Definitions are attached.

HOW TO DETERMINE IF YOU ARE BEING EXPOSED
* Exposure to hazardous substances should be routinely evaluated. This may include collecting air samples. Under OSHA 1910.20, you have a legal right to obtain copies of sampling results from your employer. If you think you are experiencing any work related health problems, see a doctor trained to recognize occupational diseases. Take this Fact Sheet with you.
* ODOR THRESHOLD = 22 ppm.
* The odor threshold only serves as a warning of exposure. Not smelling it does not mean you are not being exposed.

WORKPLACE EXPOSURE LIMITS
OSHA: The legal airborne permissible exposure limit (PEL) is 400 ppm averaged over an 8 hour work shift.

NIOSH: The recommended airborne exposure limit is 400 ppm averaged over a 10 hour work shift and 800 ppm, not to be exceeded during any 15 minute work period.
ACGIH: The recommended airborne exposure limit is 400 ppm averaged over an 8 hour work shift and 500 ppm as a STEL (short term exposure limit).
* The above exposure limits are for air levels only. When skin contact also occurs, you may be overexposed, even though air levels are less than the limits listed above.

WAYS OF REDUCING EXPOSURE
* Where possible, enclose operations and use local exhaust ventilation at the site of chemical release. If local exhaust ventilation or enclosure is not used, respirators should be worn.
* Wear protective work clothing.
* Wash thoroughly immediately after exposure to Isopropyl Alcohol and at the end of the work shift.
* Post hazard and warning information in the work area. In addition, as part of an ongoing education and training effort, communicate all information on the health and safety hazards of Isopropyl Alcohol to potentially exposed workers.

This Fact Sheet is a summary source of information of all potential and most severe health hazards that may result from exposure. Duration of exposure, concentration of the substance and other factors will affect your susceptibility to any of the potential effects described below.

HEALTH HAZARD INFORMATION
Acute Health Effects - The following acute (short term) health effects may occur immediately or shortly after exposure to Isopropyl Alcohol:
* It may irritate the skin, causing a rash or burning feeling on contact.
* Exposure can irritate the eyes, nose, and throat.
* Overexposure to the vapor may cause headaches, drowsiness, a loss of coordination, collapse, and death.

Chronic Health Effects - The following chronic (long term) health effects can occur at some time after exposure to Isopropyl Alcohol and can last for months or years:
Cancer Hazard
* There is an increased incidence of nasal sinus cancer in workers involved in the manufacture of Isopropyl Alcohol by the strong acid process. There is no evidence that Isopropyl Alcohol is a carcinogen.
Reproductive Hazard
* According to the information presently available to the New Jersey Department of Health, Isopropyl Alcohol has not been tested for its ability to adversely affect reproduction.
Other Long Term Effects -
* Skin exposure can cause itching, redness, and rashes in some people. Repeated or prolonged exposure can cause dryness and cracking of skin.

* This chemical has not been adequately evaluated to determine whether brain or other nerve damage could occur with repeated exposure. However, many solvents and other petroleum based chemicals have been shown to cause such damage. Effects may include reduced memory and concentration, personality changes (withdrawal, irritability), fatigue, sleep disturbances, reduced coordination, and/or effects on nerves supplying internal organs (autonomic nerves) and/or nerves to the arms and legs (weakness, "pins and needles").

MEDICAL TESTING
* There is no special test for this chemical. However, if illness occurs or overexposure is suspected, medical attention is recommended.
* Interview for brain effects, including recent memory, mood (irritability, withdrawal), concentration, headaches, malaise and altered sleep patterns. Consider cerebellar, autonomic and peripheral nervous system evaluation. Positive and borderline individuals should be referred for neuropsychological testing. Any evaluation should include a careful history of past and present symptoms with an exam. Medical tests that look for damage already done are not a substitute for controlling exposure.
Request copies of your medical testing. You have a legal right to this information under OSHA 1910.20.

WORKPLACE CONTROLS AND PRACTICES
Unless a less toxic chemical can be substituted for a hazardous substance, ENGINEERING CONTROLS are the most effective way of reducing exposure. The best protection is to enclose operations and/or provide local exhaust ventilation at the site of chemical release. Isolating operations can also reduce exposure. Using respirators or protective equipment is less effective than the controls mentioned above, but is sometimes necessary.
In evaluating the controls present in your workplace, consider: (1) how hazardous the substance is, (2) how much of the substance is released into the workplace and (3) whether harmful skin or eye contact could occur. Special controls should be in place for highly toxic chemicals or when significant skin, eye, or breathing exposures are possible. In addition, the following controls are recommended:
* Where possible, automatically pump liquid Isopropyl Alcohol from drums or other storage containers to process containers.
* Specific engineering controls are recommended for this chemical by NIOSH. Refer to the NIOSH criteria document: Isopropyl Alcohol #76 142.
Good WORK PRACTICES can help to reduce hazardous exposures. The following work practices are recommended:
* Workers whose clothing has been contaminated by Isopropyl Alcohol should change into clean clothing promptly.
* Contaminated work clothes should be laundered by individuals who have been informed of the hazards of exposure to Isopropyl Alcohol.

* On skin contact with Isopropyl Alcohol, immediately wash or shower to remove the chemical. At the end of the work shift, wash any areas of the body that may have contacted Isopropyl Alcohol, whether or not known skin contact has occurred.

* Do not eat, smoke, or drink where Isopropyl Alcohol is handled, processed, or stored, since the chemical can be swallowed. Wash hands carefully before eating or smoking.

PERSONAL PROTECTIVE EQUIPMENT
WORKPLACE CONTROLS ARE BETTER THAN PERSONAL PROTECTIVE EQUIPMENT. However, for some jobs (such as outside work, confined space entry, jobs done only once in a while, or jobs done while workplace controls are being installed), personal protective equipment may be appropriate. The following recommendations are only guidelines and may not apply to every situation.

Clothing

* Avoid skin contact with Isopropyl Alcohol. Wear solvent resistant gloves and clothing. Safety equipment suppliers/manufacturers can provide recommendations on the most protective glove/ clothing material for your operation.

* All protective clothing (suits, gloves, footwear, headgear) should be clean, available each day, and put on before work.

* ACGIH recommends natural rubber, neoprene, nitrile, or polyvinyl chloride protective material.

Eye Protection

* Wear splash proof chemical goggles and face shield when working with liquid, unless full face piece respiratory protection is worn.

Respiratory Protection

IMPROPER USE OF RESPIRATORS IS DANGEROUS. Such equipment should only be used if the employer has a written program that takes into account workplace conditions, requirements for worker training, respirator fit testing and medical exams, as described in OSHA 1910.134.

* Where the potential exists for exposures near or over 400 ppm, use a MSHA/ NIOSH approved respirator with an organic vapor cartridge/canister. More protection is provided by a full face piece respirator than by a half mask respirator, and even greater protection is provided by a powered air purifying respirator.

* If while wearing a filter, cartridge or canister respirator, you can smell, taste, or otherwise detect Isopropyl Alcohol, or in the case of a full face piece respirator you experience eye irritation, leave the area immediately. Check to make sure the respirator to face seal is still good. If it is, replace the filter, cartridge, or canister. If the seal is no longer good, you may need a new respirator.

* Be sure to consider all potential exposures in your workplace. You may need a combination of filters, prefilters, cartridges, or canisters to protect against different forms of a chemical (such as vapor and mist) or against a mixture of chemicals.

* Where the potential for higher exposures exists, use a MSHA/NIOSH approved supplied air respirator with a full face piece operated in the positive pressure mode or with a full face piece, hood, or helmet in the continuous flow mode, or use a

MSHA/NIOSH approved self contained breathing apparatus with a full face piece operated in pressure demand or other positive pressure mode.
* Exposure to 20,000 ppm is immediately dangerous to life and health. If the possibility of exposures above 20,000 ppm exists, use a MSHA/NIOSH approved self contained breathing apparatus with a full face piece operated in continuous flow or other positive pressure mode.

HANDLING AND STORAGE
* Prior to working with Isopropyl Alcohol you should be trained on its proper handling and storage.
* Isopropyl Alcohol must be stored to avoid contact with STRONG OXIDIZERS (such as CHLORINE, BROMINE, and FLUORINE) since violent reactions occur.
* Store in tightly closed containers in a cool, well ventilated area away from HEAT.
* Sources of ignition, such as smoking and open flames, are prohibited where Isopropyl Alcohol is used, handled, or stored in a manner that could create a potential fire or explosion hazard.
* Metal containers involving the transfer of 5 gallons or more of Isopropyl Alcohol should be grounded and bonded. Drums must be equipped with self closing valves, pressure vacuum bungs, and flame arresters.
* Use only non sparking tools and equipment, especially when opening and closing containers of Isopropyl Alcohol.

Common Name: Isopropyl Alcohol   DOT Number: UN 1219
DOT Emergency Guide code: 26   CAS Number: 67-63-0
Hazard rating   NJ DOH NFPA
FLAMMABILITY   -   3
REACTIVITY   -   0
POISONOUS GASES ARE PRODUCED IN FIRE
CONTAINERS MAY EXPLODE IN FIRE
Hazard Rating Key: 0=minimal; 1=slight; 2=moderate; 3=serious; 4=severe

FIRE HAZARDS
* Isopropyl Alcohol is a FLAMMABLE LIQUID.
* Vapors may travel to a source of ignition and flash back.
* CONTAINERS MAY EXPLODE IN FIRE.
* Use dry chemical, CO2, water spray, or alcohol foam extinguishers.
* POISONOUS GASES ARE PRODUCED IN FIRE.
* If employees are expected to fight fires, they must be trained and equipped as stated in OSHA 1910.156.

SPILLS AND EMERGENCIES
If Isopropyl Alcohol is spilled or leaked, take the following steps:

* Restrict persons not wearing protective equipment from area of spill or leak until cleanup is complete.
* Remove all ignition sources.
* Ventilate area of spill or leak.
* Absorb liquids in vermiculite, dry sand, earth, or a similar material and deposit in sealed containers.
* Keep Isopropyl Alcohol out of a confined space, such as a sewer, because of the possibility of an explosion, unless the sewer is designed to prevent the buildup of explosive concentrations.
* It may be necessary to contain and dispose of Isopropyl Alcohol as a HAZARDOUS WASTE. Contact your Department of Environmental Protection (DEP) or your regional office of the federal Environmental Protection Agency (EPA) for specific recommendations.

FOR LARGE SPILLS AND FIRES immediately call your fire department.

FIRST AID
POISON INFORMATION
Eye Contact
* Immediately flush with large amounts of water for at least 15 minutes, occasionally lifting upper and lower lids.
Skin Contact
* Quickly remove contaminated clothing. Immediately wash contaminated skin with large amounts of water.
Breathing
* Remove the person from exposure.
* Begin rescue breathing if breathing has stopped and CPR if heart action has stopped.
* Transfer promptly to a medical facility.

PHYSICAL DATA
Vapor Pressure: 33 mm Hg at 68°F (20°C)
Flash Point: 53°F (11.6°C)
Water Solubility: Miscible

OTHER COMMONLY USED NAMES
Chemical Name: 2-Propanol
Other Names and Formulations: Rubbing Alcohol; Dimethylcarbinol; Isopropanol; sec-Propyl Alcohol.

NEW JERSEY DEPARTMENT OF HEALTH
Right to Know Program   CN 368,   Trenton, NJ 08625 0368

ECOLOGICAL INFORMATION

Isopropyl alcohol is a clear, flammable liquid with numerous uses. It is used in antifreeze; as a solvent for gums, shellac and essential oils; in quick-drying inks and oils; in cosmetics such as body rubs, hand lotions and after-shave lotions; and to make other chemicals. It may enter the environment from industrial discharges, municipal waste water treatment discharges, or spills.

ACUTE (SHORT-TERM) ECOLOGICAL EFFECTS
Acute toxic effects may include the death of animals, birds, or fish, and death or low growth rate in plants. Acute effects are seen two to four days after animals or plants come in contact with a toxic chemical substance. Isopropyl alcohol has slight toxicity to aquatic life. Insufficient data are available to evaluate or predict the short-term effects of isopropyl alcohol to plants, birds, or land animals.

CHRONIC (LONG-TERM) ECOLOGICAL EFFECTS
Chronic toxic effects may include shortened lifespan, reproductive problems, lower fertility, and changes in appearance or behavior. Chronic effects can be seen long after first exposure(s) to a toxic chemical. Isopropyl alcohol has slight chronic toxicity to aquatic organisms. Insufficient data are available to evaluate or predict the long- term effects of isopropyl alcohol to plants, birds, or land animals.

WATER SOLUBILITY
Isopropyl alcohol is highly soluble in water. Concentrations of 1,000 milligrams and more will mix with a liter of water.

DISTRIBUTION AND PERSISTENCE IN THE ENVIRONMENT
Isopropyl alcohol is slightly persistent in water, with a half-life of between 2 to 20 days. The half-life of a pollutant is the amount of time it takes for one-half of the chemical to be degraded. About 77.5% of isopropyl alcohol will eventually end up in water; the rest will end up in the air.

BIOACCUMULATION IN AQUATIC ORGANISMS
Some substances increase in concentration, or bioaccumulate, in living organisms as they breathe contaminated air, drink contaminated water, or eat contaminated food. These chemicals can become concentrated in the tissues and internal organs of animals and humans. The concentration of isopropyl alcohol found in fish tissues is expected to be about the same as the average concentration of isopropyl alcohol in the water from which the fish was taken.

SUPPORT DOCUMENT: AQUIRE Database, ERL-Duluth, U.S. EPA, Phytotox.

(source: **gopher://ecosys.drdr.Virginia.edu:70/11/library/gen/toxics**)

HAZARD COMMUNICATION PROGRAM EXAMPLE

Established For:_____
_____(Name and Address of practice)

In compliance with OSHA Hazard Communication Rules (29 CFR 1910.1200), and in the interest of illness and injury prevention, the management staff of this practice is required to provide a safe and healthful workplace. All levels of supervision are accountable for the health and safety of employees under their direction, and share responsibility for hazard communications pursuant to this written program.

This written program will be located in:_____
and is available for review by any interested employees. Additionally, copies will be given to all current and new employees. We will meet the requirements of this rule as follows:

Container Labeling
_____(Name & Title of person responsible) will verify that all containers of hazardous chemicals will: be clearly labeled as to contents; supply appropriate hazard warnings; and list manufacturer's name and address.

Secondary containers will be labeled with a copy of the original manufacturer's label, or with generic labels with identification and hazard warning information. It is company policy that no containers of chemicals will be used without such labeling.
_____(Name & Title of person responsible) will ensure that all secondary containers are labeled with chemical identification and hazard warnings.

Material Safety Data Sheets (MSDS's)
Copies of MSDS's for all hazardous chemicals to which employees may be exposed will be kept in:_____.
MSDS's will be available to all employees in their work area for review during each work shift. If MSDS's are not available for a chemical in use, immediately contact:
_____ (Name & Title of person responsible).

Employee Information & Training
Prior to starting work, each of our new employees will attend a health and safety orientation and will receive information and training on the following:
* Overview of requirements of Hazard Communication Rules 29CFR1910.1200;
* Chemicals present in our workplace operations;
* location and availability of our written hazard communication program;
* Physical and health effects of the hazardous chemicals;

* Methods and observation techniques used to determine the presence or release of hazardous chemicals in the work area;
* Ways to reduce or prevent exposure through work practices and personal protective equipment;
* Other steps we have taken to reduce or prevent exposure;
* Emergency procedures to follow for hazardous exposures; and
* How to read labels and review MSDS's to obtain hazard information.

After attending training class, each employee will sign a form to verify that they attended, received our written materials, and understood our company policies on hazard communication.

Prior to a new hazardous chemical being introduced in our workplace, each at risk employee will be given information as outlined above. _____

(Name & Title of person responsible) is responsible for ensuring that MSDS's of new chemicals are available.

Hazardous Chemicals List

The following is a list of all known hazardous chemicals used by our employees. More information on each chemical is located in the MSDS file, referenced above.

HAZARDOUS CHEMICAL	MAX.AMT.	LOCATION	USES
1. Isopropyl Alcohol	1 gal.	Cabinet A	SkinDisinfectant
2. Bleach	1 gal.	Cabinet B	Cleaning
Etc.			

(Update list as new hazardous chemicals enter workplace)

Hazardous Non-Routine Tasks

If there are ever hazardous non-routine tasks, before starting work on such projects, each affected employee will be given information by their supervisor about the hazardous chemicals to which they may be exposed during such activity. The information will include: Specific chemical hazards; Protective and safety measures; Other measures we have taken to reduce hazards (including ventilation, presence of another employee, and emergency procedures). Note: Our company does not transfer chemicals through pipes.

Informing Contractors

When contractors are on site in our workplace, _____
(Name & Title of person responsible) is responsible for providing them with the following information: Hazardous chemicals to which they may be exposed; Procedures for obtaining MSDS's; Precautions and protective measures employees may use; and an explanation of our labeling system. The aforementioned responsible person will also identify and obtain MSDS's for hazardous chemicals the contractor brings into our workplace.

Date of Initial Plan:_____   Reviewed & Updated:_____

HEPATITIS B VACCINE DECLINATION FORM

29 CFR 1910.1030 App. A

I understand that due to my occupational exposure to blood or other potentially infectious materials I may be at risk of acquiring hepatitis B virus (HBV) infection. I have been given the opportunity to be vaccinated with hepatitis B vaccine, at no charge to myself. However, I decline hepatitis B vaccination at this time. I understand that by declining this vaccine, I continue to be at risk of acquiring hepatitis B, a serious disease. If in the future I continue to have occupational exposure to blood or other potentially infectious materials and I want to be vaccinated with hepatitis B vaccine, I can receive the vaccination series at no charge to me.

Employee:_____

Date:_____

Employer:_____

Note: use of the above wording is mandatory.

EMPLOYEE MEDICAL RECORD

CONFIDENTIAL- REQUIRE EMPLOYEE'S WRITTEN PERMISSION FOR RELEASE

Employer & Site:_____

Employee:_____ SSN:_____

Job Title:_____ Date Hired:_____

Date Employment Ended:_____

HBV Vaccination Status:_____

HBV Vaccination Dates:_____, _____, _____

If HBV Vaccine declined, is Declination Form signed?   Yes   No

HBV Antibody Test Results: Pos.   Neg.   Not Taken   Test Date_____

TB PPD Test Results: Pos.   Neg.   Not Taken   Test Date_____

(Attach documentation of vaccination, exempt status, declination form, and any records related to ability to receive vaccine. Attach documentation of all post-exposure evaluation & follow-up.)

EXPOSURE INCIDENT HISTORY

Incident #1:

Date & Time of Incident: _____

Date Information Supplied to Healthcare Professional: _____

Date Healthcare Professional's Written Opinion Filed:_____

Date Post Exposure Evaluation Record Filed:_____

RETAIN THIS RECORD FOR 30 YEARS FROM TERMINATION OF EMPLOYMENT

SAMPLE EMPLOYEE MEDICAL RECORDS RELEASE FORM

29 CFR 1910.1020 App. A - Non-Mandatory Guideline

I, _____, (full name of worker/patient) hereby authorize _____ (individual or organization holding the medical records) to release to _____ (individual or organization authorized to receive the medical information), the following medical information from my personal medical records: _____

_____

(Describe generally the information desired to be released)

I give my permission for this medical information to be used for the following purpose:

_____

but I do not give permission for any other use or re-disclosure of this information.

(Note: several extra lines are provided below so that you can place additional restrictions on this authorization letter if you want to. You may, however, leave these lines blank. On the other hand, you may want to (1) specify a particular expiration date for this letter (if less than one year); (2) describe medical information to be created in the future that you intend to be covered by this authorization letter; or (3) describe portions of the medical information in your records which you do not intend to be released as a result of this letter.)

_____

_____

Full name of Employee or Legal Representative

_____

Signature of Employee or Legal Representative

_____

Date of Signature

[61 FR 31427, June 20, 1996]

EMPLOYER'S EXPOSURE INCIDENT REPORT

CONFIDENTIAL -REQUIRE EMPLOYEE'S WRITTEN PERMISSION FOR RELEASE

Employer & Site:_____

Employee:_____ SSN:_____

Job Title:_____

Date & Time of Incident:_____

Route(s) of Exposure: _____

Job Duties Related to Exposure Incident:_____
_____

Description of Exposure Incident :_____
_____
_____

Source Individual Involved & How to Contact:(include NO confidential info about source)
_____

Source Individual HIV and HBV infectious status already known?   Yes   No
Source Individual Consent for Testing Obtained?   Yes   No   Date:_____
Source Referred for Testing to: Dr._____ Date:_____

Suggested changes in work practices & policies to prevent future occurrences:
_____
_____

Date changes completed:_____

Signature of Employee:_____ Date:_____

Signature Exposure Control Plan Admin:_____ Date:_____

Employee Referred to the following Healthcare Professional for Post Exposure Medical Evaluation: Dr._____ Date:_____

HEALTHCARE PROFESSIONAL'S
POST EXPOSURE WRITTEN OPINION

CONFIDENTIAL - REQUIRE EMPLOYEE'S WRITTEN PERMISSION FOR RELEASE

Employer & Site:_____

Employee:_____ SSN:_____

Job Title:_____

EMPLOYER: Attach Employee Medical Record; Exposure Incident Report; and a Copy of 29CFR1910.1030; convey to healthcare professional doing post-exposure evaluation.

Our employee has been referred to you due to an occupational exposure to blood or other potentially infectious material. Please provide the following information:

Employee has been informed of results of my evaluation and any exposure related conditions.   Date_____

Hepatitis B Vaccine indicated?   Yes   No   Vaccination Dates:_____

Employee has been told about any medical condition resulting from blood or OPIM which require further evaluation or treatment.   Date:_____

Physician Signature/Date_____

Employee Signature/Date:_____

POST EXPOSURE EVALUATION RECORD

CONFIDENTIAL - RELEASE ONLY WITH EMPLOYEE'S WRITTEN PERMISSION AND AFTER INFORMING EMPLOYEE OF CONFIDENTIALITY REQUIREMENTS REGARDING SOURCE INDIVIDUAL INFORMATION

Employer & Site:_____

Employee:_____ SSN:_____

Job Title:_____ Exposure Incident Date:_____

Identity of Source Individual:_____
Consent for Source Individual's Blood Testing Obtained: Yes   No
Date:_____   If No, Reason:_____
Source Individual Referred To: Dr._____ Date:_____
Are Source Individual's HIV & HBV Infectivity Status known to Employer, making further testing unnecessary?   Yes   No
If Yes, date this infomation was conveyed to Post Exposure Physician: _____

Have Source Individual HIV & HBV Test Results Been Provided to Employee by Physician?   Yes   No   Date_____ **Employee Initials**_____

Employee informed of laws & regulations concerning disclosure of identity and infectious status of source individual. Date:_____ **Employee Initials**_____

Date Exposure Incident Report Filed:_____

Date Employee Referred to Healthcare Professional for Evaluation:_____

Employee Referred To: Dr._____

Date(s) Post Exposure Prophylaxis Provided:_____, _____, _____

Date Counseling Offered:_____ Referred To_____

Date Healthcare Professional's Post-Exposure Written Opinion Obtained:_____

Healthcare Professional's Post-Exposure Written Opinion Provided to Employee On Date:_____ **Employee Initials**_____

BLOODBORNE PATHOGENS EXPOSURE CONTROL PLAN EXAMPLE

Facility Name: _____

The management staff of the above named facility are committed to the prevention of employee injury and illness caused by bloodborne pathogen exposure incidents. In compliance with OSHA Bloodborne Pathogens Standard 29 CFR 1910.1030, we hereby adopt this Exposure Control Plan (ECP) as an element of our Safety and Health Program.

A. Purposes
To eliminate or minimize employee occupational exposure to blood or other potentially infectious materials (OPIM);
To identify employees at risk of occupational exposure to blood or OPIM while performing their regular job duties;
To provide training and information to employees at risk of occupational exposure to blood or OPIM. A copy of this plan is available to all employees during work shifts, in the following location: _____.
To comply with OSHA Bloodborne Pathogen Standard 29 CFR 1910.1030.

B. Exposure Determination
Our facility has performed an exposure determination, identifying job classifications for which every employee in the classification may be expected to incur occupational exposures to blood or OPIM. Exposure determination was made without regard to use of PPE. The following job classifications are in this category:

1. ACUPUNCTURIST

In the following job classifications, <u>some</u> of the employees may have occupational blood or OPIM exposure risks. At risk tasks and procedures have been identified.

Job Classification	Task / Procedure

NONE (assumes Acupuncturist does all housekeeping, handles all contam. & reg. waste, contam. laundry, decontamination chores, and first aid provision)

C. Compliance Methods
1. Universal Precautions:
'Universal precautions' is an approach to infection control that requires employers and employees to assume that all human blood and specified body fluids are infectious for

HIV, HBV and other bloodborne pathogens. Where differentiation of types of body fluids is difficult, all body fluids are considered to be potentially infectious.

2. Engineering Controls and Work Practices:
Engineering and work practice controls will be used by all employees to eliminate or minimize occupational exposure incidents at this facility.

The **engineering controls** are:
a. Contaminated sharps will be disposed of in red plastic sharps containers located in close proximity to sharps use area. Sharps containers shall be maintained upright throughout use, replaced routinely, and not be allowed to overfill.

The **work practices** are:
a. Wash hands and any other skin with soap and water, or flush mucous membranes with water immediately or as soon as feasible following contact of such body areas with blood or OPIM.
b. Wash hands immediately or as soon as feasible after removal of gloves or other PPE.
c. Contaminated needles shall not be bent, sheared or broken.
d. Contaminated sharps shall be discarded immediately or as soon as feasible in red plastic sharps containers.
e. Sharps containers, when moved, will be closed immediately prior to removal.
f. Eating, drinking, smoking, applying cosmetics or lip balm, and contact lens handling are prohibited in work areas where there is likelihood of occupational exposure.
g. All needles and coining friction devices will be single use disposables.
h. Cupping jars will be disposed of immediately or as soon as feasible after a use in which they contact blood or OPIM.
I. All procedures involving blood or OPIM shall be performed in such a manner as to minimize splashing, spraying, spattering and generation of droplets of these substances.
j. Broken glassware which may be contaminated shall not be picked up directly with the hands. Use brush and dustpan, and tongs or forceps.

3. Personal Protective Equipment (PPE):
The following PPE will be provided at no cost to employees:
(LIST ITEMS AND WHEN TO BE USED)

a. Body Protection: Not Needed. Lab coats may be worn as professional uniforms, and are not intended to be PPE at our facility.

b. Gloves and Masks: Disposable latex examination gloves will be used on both hands for all Coining procedures; for Cupping procedures when blood is drawn into the suction cups; for Bloodletting at acupuncture points; for Acupoint Injections; whenever there is hand contact with mucous membranes or non-intact skin; whenever there is hand contact with blood or OPIM; and whenever the employee has cuts, scratches or other breaks in the skin of their hands. When acupuncture needles are removed, at a minimum, the one hand holding the cotton ball for compression at the sites must be gloved. Re-useable rubber utility gloves will be used on both hands for all cleaning of equipment and environmental surfaces; for handling of contaminated and red-bagged regulated waste containers; for handling of contaminated laundry; and for cleanup of broken glass. Disposable resuscitation barriers will be used for CPR procedures, unless a ventilation bag is available.

c. Eye Protection: None needed. (Laser protective eyewear if Class IIIb Lasers are used)

d. Special PPE: None needed.

The following person is responsible to issue appropriate and readily accessible PPE, without cost, to employees:_____(Name, Job Title) Low-protein latex gloves, powderless gloves, or other alternatives will be readily accessible to employees allergic to gloves normally provided.

All PPE will be removed prior to leaving the work area.

All PPE will be cleaned, laundered and disposed of by the employer, at no cost to the employee.

Removed PPE (other than disposable PPE) will be placed in the following location for storage, washing, decontamination, inspection, an/or disposal:
_____.

4. Housekeeping:
This facility will be cleaned and decontaminated according to the following schedule:

AREA	SCHEDULE	PROCEDURE
sinks, countertops, work surfaces	end of each shift and whenever visibly contaminated	Bleach sol. 1:10 - 1:100 Rubber utility glove PPE
waste containers in treatment areas	weekly and whenever visibly contaminated	Bleach sol. 1:10 - 1:100 Rubber utility glove PPE Replace plastic bag liner
floors	weekly and whenever visibly contaminated	Vacuum clean; Damp mop as needed Bleach sol. as needed w/ Rubber utility glove PPE

5. Contaminated Laundry:

Contaminated laundry will be handled minimally, bagged and labeled biohazardous. Contaminated laundry will be cleaned at the following location: _____

NOTE: This facility does not normally produce any contaminated laundry.

6. Regulated Waste:

The following procedures will be followed:

a. Sharps containers shall be closable, puncture resistant, leakproof on sides and bottom, biohazard labeled, red in color, and closed prior to removal.

b. Other regulated waste shall be red-bagged, protectively stored, and sealed closed prior to removal.

c. Disposal of all regulated waste shall be in accordance with federal, state and local regulations.

7. HBV Vaccine and Post-Exposure Evaluation and Follow-up:
   HBV Vaccine

The HBV vaccination series for employees at risk, and post-exposure evaluation, care and follow-up will be provided at: (Name, Phone Number, & Location of Healthcare Provider)_____
_____.

The person responsible for our HBV vaccination program is:_____
_____(Name, Job Title). They will ensure that all medical evaluations and procedures, including HBV vaccination, post-exposure evaluation, lab tests, care, prophylaxis, and follow-up are made available at no charge to the employee, at a reasonable time and place, and performed by a licensed healthcare provider according to then current USPHS recommendations. Employees declining HBV vaccination will be required to sign the OSHA HBV vaccine declination form. Employee's declination does not preclude their option to later accept and receive vaccination. Participation in pre-screening will not be a prerequisite for receiving HBV vaccination.

HBV vaccination shall be made available to all employees at risk of occupational exposure, after employee has received training (see 9. below) and within 10 days of initial assignment, unless employee has completed the vaccination series previously, is proven immune by antibody testing, or the vaccine is medically contraindicated. If booster doses are later recommended by USPHS, they shall also be made available.

   Post Exposure Evaluation and Follow-up

When an employee has an exposure incident, it will be immediately reported to: _____(Name, Job Title).

With report of an exposure incident, the employer will make available to the exposed employee a confidential medical evaluation and follow-up with at least the following elements:

Documentation of routes of exposure, and circumstances of exposure incident;

Identification of the source individual unless infeasible or legally prohibited;

Prompt testing of source individual's blood to determine HIV and HBV infectivity (if legal to do), if consent can be obtained, or establishment that consent cannot be obtained. If source individual is already known to be HIV or HBV infected, testing need not be repeated.

Results of source individual's testing shall be made available to exposed employee, and employee informed of confidentiality concerning disclosure of source individual's name and infectious status;

Prompt testing, upon consent, of employee's blood for HBV and HIV serological status; If employee consents to baseline blood testing but declines HIV testing, the blood sample will be preserved at least 90 days to secure employee's option to consent to HIV testing.

Post-exposure prophylaxis as recommended by USPHS;

Counseling; and

Evaluation of reported illnesses.

Information Provided to Healthcare Professional

_____(Name, Job Title) will ensure that the healthcare professional responsible for the employee's HBV vaccination and for post-exposure evaluation, care and follow-up, is provided with the following:

A copy of 29CFR1910.1030;

Description of employee's duties as related to exposure incident;

Documentation of routes of exposure and circumstances of exposure incident;

Results of source individual's blood testing, if available; and

All employee medical records relevant to employee's appropriate treatment, including vaccination status.

Healthcare Professional's Written Opinion

_____(Name, Job Title) will obtain and provide the employee with a copy of the healthcare professional's post-exposure written opinion, within 15 days of completion of that medical evaluation.

The healthcare professional's written opinion regarding HBV vaccination will be limited to whether vaccination is indicated for an employee, and if it has been given.

The healthcare professional's written opinion regarding post-exposure follow-up shall be limited to the following information:

That the employee has been informed of the results of the examination;

That the employee has been told about any medical conditions resulting from exposure to blood or OPIM which require further evaluation or treatment.

Diagnoses and other findings shall remain confidential and shall not be included in the report.

8. Labels and Signs:
The following person is responsible for ensuring that biohazard labels are on each container of regulated waste, and/or that said waste is in a red-colored protective container: (Name, Job Title)_____.
Sharps containers and red plastic bags are our usual regulated waste containers.

9. Information and Training:
The following person is responsible for ensuring that training is provided at time of initial employee assignment to tasks with risks of occupational exposure, and that training will be repeated within 12 month intervals: (Name, Job Title)_____
_____.
Training will be tailored to education and language level of employees, and offered during normal work shift hours. It will contain at a minimum the following informational and interactional elements:
An accessible copy of 29CFR1910.1030 and an explanation of its contents;
General explanation of epidemiology and symptoms of bloodborne diseases;
Explanation of modes of transmission of bloodborne pathogens;
An accessible copy of this Exposure Control Plan, and explanation of its contents;
Explanation of appropriate methods for recognizing tasks with risk of blood or OPIM exposure;
Explanation of use and limits of risk reduction methods, including engineering controls, work practices and PPE;
Information on types, proper use, location, removal, handling, decontamination and disposal of PPE;
Explanation of basis for selection of PPE;
Information on HBV vaccine, including efficacy, safety, method of administration, benefits, and availability without charge;
Appropriate actions and persons to contact in an emergency involving blood or OPIM;
Procedure to follow if an exposure incident occurs, including method of reporting incident and the medical follow-up that will be made available;
Information on post-exposure evaluation and follow-up required to be provided by employer;
Explanation of biohazard signs, labels and color coding;
Opportunity for interactive questions and answers with person conducting training session.

Trainer shall be knowledgeable in the subject matter as it relates to acupuncture. Additional training will be given to employees when there are task or procedure changes affecting employee occupational exposure.

10. Recordkeeping:

The following person is responsible for maintaining employee medical records: (Name, Job Title) _____.

These records will be kept at: _____(location), and will be maintained for 30 years beyond the duration of employment. The employer shall ensure that medical records are kept confidential, requiring the employee's written authorization for release, unless release is otherwise mandated. Employees may request and receive copies of their own medical record.

The employee medical record will include:

Name and social security number of employee;

Employee's HBV vaccination status, dates of HBV vaccinations, and any medical records relative to employee's ability to receive vaccination;

Copy of results of examinations, medical testing and follow-up procedures required in post-exposure evaluation and follow-up;

Employer's copy of healthcare professional's post exposure written opinion; and

Copy of the information provided to the healthcare professional.

11. Training Records:

The following person is responsible for maintaining bloodborne pathogen training records: (Name, Job Title)_____.

These records will be kept at: _____(location), and will be maintained for 3 years from the date of the training.

Training records will include:

Dates of training sessions;

Contents or summary of training sessions;

Names and qualifications of persons conducting the training; and

Names and job titles of persons attending the training sessions.

D. Evaluation and Review:

_____(Name, Job Title) is responsible for reviewing this Exposure Control Plan annually or as needed, and updating as needed.

Exposure Control Program has been Adopted on this date:_____,
By_____ (highest mgmnt. official)

Records of reviews and updates will be appended.

APPENDIX B

HAZARD COMMUNICATION
29 CFR 1910.1200

(a) Purpose. (1) The purpose of this section is to ensure that the hazards of all chemicals produced or imported are evaluated, and that information concerning their hazards is transmitted to employers and employees. This transmittal of information is to be accomplished by means of comprehensive hazard communication programs, which are to include container labeling and other forms of warning, material safety data sheets and employee training. (2) This occupational safety and health standard is intended to address comprehensively the issue of evaluating the potential hazards of chemicals, and communicating information concerning hazards and appropriate protective measures to employees, and to preempt any legal requirements of a state, or political subdivision of a state, pertaining to this subject. Evaluating the potential hazards of chemicals, and communicating information concerning hazards and appropriate protective measures to employees, may include, for example, but is not limited to, provisions for: developing and maintaining a written hazard communication program for the workplace, including lists of hazardous chemicals present; labeling of containers of chemicals in the workplace, as well as of containers of chemicals being shipped to other workplaces; preparation and distribution of material safety data sheets to employees and downstream employers; and development and implementation of employee training programs regarding hazards of chemicals and protective measures. Under section 18 of the Act, no state or political subdivision of a state may adopt or enforce, through any court or agency, any requirement relating to the issue addressed by this Federal standard, except pursuant to a Federally-approved state plan.

(b) Scope and application. (1) This section requires chemical manufacturers or importers to assess the hazards of chemicals which they produce or import, and all employers to provide information to their employees about the hazardous chemicals to which they are exposed, by means of a hazard communication program, labels and other forms of warning, material safety data sheets, and information and training. In addition, this section requires distributors to transmit the required information to employers. (Employers who do not produce or import chemicals need only focus on those parts of this rule that deal with establishing a workplace program and communicating information to their workers. Appendix E of this section is a general guide for such employers to help them determine their compliance obligations under the rule.) (2) This section applies to any chemical which is known to be present in the workplace in such a manner that employees may be exposed under normal conditions of use or in a foreseeable emergency. (3) This section applies to laboratories only as follows: (I) Employers shall ensure that labels on incoming containers of hazardous chemicals are not removed or defaced; (ii)

Employers shall maintain any material safety data sheets that are received with incoming shipments of hazardous chemicals, and ensure that they are readily accessible during each work shift to laboratory employees when they are in their work areas; (iii) Employers shall ensure that laboratory employees are provided information and training in accordance with paragraph (h) of this section, except for the location and availability of the written hazard communication program under paragraph (h)(2)(iii) of this section; and, (iv) Laboratory employers that ship hazardous chemicals are considered to be either a chemical manufacturer or a distributor under this rule, and thus must ensure that any containers of hazardous chemicals leaving the laboratory are labeled in accordance with paragraph (f)(1) of this section, and that a material safety data sheet is provided to distributors and other employers in accordance with paragraphs (g)(6) and (g)(7) of this section. (4) In work operations where employees only handle chemicals in sealed containers which are not opened under normal conditions of use (such as are found in marine cargo handling, warehousing, or retail sales), this section applies to these operations only as follows: (I) Employers shall ensure that labels on incoming containers of hazardous chemicals are not removed or defaced; (ii) Employers shall maintain copies of any material safety data sheets that are received with incoming shipments of the sealed containers of hazardous chemicals, shall obtain a material safety data sheet as soon as possible for sealed containers of hazardous chemicals received without a material safety data sheet if an employee requests the material safety data sheet, and shall ensure that the material safety data sheets are readily accessible during each work shift to employees when they are in their work area(s);and, (iii) Employers shall ensure that employees are provided with information and training in accordance with paragraph (h) of this section (except for the location and availability of the written hazard communication program under paragraph (h)(2)(iii) of this section), to the extent necessary to protect them in the event of a spill or leak of a hazardous chemical from a sealed container. (5) This section does not require labeling of the following chemicals: (I) Any pesticide as such term is defined in the Federal Insecticide, Fungicide, and Rodenticide Act (7 U.S.C. 136 et seq.), when subject to the labeling requirements of that Act and labeling regulations issued under that Act by the Environmental Protection Agency; (ii) Any chemical substance or mixture as such terms are defined in the Toxic Substances Control Act (15 U.S.C. 2601 et seq.), when subject to the labeling requirements of that Act and labeling regulations issued under that Act by the Environmental Protection Agency. (iii) Any food, food additive, color additive, drug, cosmetic, or medical or veterinary device or product, including materials intended for use as ingredients in such products (e.g. flavors and fragrances), as such terms are defined in the Federal Food, Drug, and Cosmetic Act (21 U.S.C. 301 et seq.) or the Virus-Serum-Toxin Act of 1913 (21 U.S.C. 151 et seq.), and regulations issued under those Acts, when they are subject to the labeling requirements under those Acts by either the Food and Drug Administration or the Department of Agriculture; (iv) Any distilled spirits (beverage alcohols), wine, or malt beverage intended for nonindustrial use, as such terms are defined in the Federal Alcohol Administration Act (27 U.S.C. 201 et seq.) and regulations issued under that Act, when subject to the labeling requirements of that Act and labeling regulations issued under that Act by the

Appendix B Hazard Communication   283

Bureau of Alcohol, Tobacco, and Firearms; (v) Any consumer product or hazardous substance as those terms are defined in the Consumer Product Safety Act (15 U.S.C. 2051 et seq.) and Federal Hazardous Substances Act (15 U.S.C. 1261 et seq.) respectively, when subject to a consumer product safety standard or labeling requirement of those Acts, or regulations issued under those Acts by the Consumer Product Safety Commission; and, (vi) Agricultural or vegetable seed treated with pesticides and labeled in accordance with the Federal Seed Act (7 U.S.C. 1551 et seq.) and the labeling regulations issued under that Act by the Department of Agriculture. (6) This section does not apply to: (I) Any hazardous waste as such term is defined by the Solid Waste Disposal Act, as amended by the Resource Conservation and Recovery Act of 1976, as amended (42 U.S.C. 6901 et seq.), when subject to regulations issued under that Act by the Environmental Protection Agency; (ii) Any hazardous substance as such term is defined by the Comprehensive Environmental Response, Compensation and Liability ACT (CERCLA) (42 U.S.C. 9601 et seq.) when the hazardous substance is the focus of remedial or removal action being conducted under CERCLA in accordance with Environmental Protection Agency regulations; (iii) Tobacco or tobacco products; (iv) Wood or wood products, including lumber which will not be processed, where the chemical manufacturer or importer can establish that the only hazard they pose to employees is the potential for flammability or combustibility (wood or wood products which have been treated with a hazardous chemical covered by this standard, and wood which may be subsequently sawed or cut, generating dust, are not exempted); (v) Articles (as that term is defined in paragraph C of this section); (vi) Food or alcoholic beverages which are sold, used, or prepared in a retail establishment (such as a grocery store, restaurant, or drinking place), and foods intended for personal consumption by employees while in the workplace; (vii) Any drug, as that term is defined in the Federal Food, Drug, and Cosmetic Act (21 U.S.C. 301 et seq.), when it is in solid, final form for direct administration to the patient (e.g., tablets or pills); drugs which are packaged by the chemical manufacturer for sale to consumers in a retail establishment (e.g., over-the-counter drugs); and drugs intended for personal consumption by employees while in the workplace (e.g., first aid supplies); (viii) Cosmetics which are packaged for sale to consumers in a retail establishment, and cosmetics intended for personal consumption by employees while in the workplace; (ix) Any consumer product or hazardous substance, as those terms are defined in the Consumer Product Safety Act (15 U.S.C. 2051 et seq.) and Federal Hazardous Substances Act (15 U.S.C. 1261 et seq.) respectively, where the employer can show that it is used in the workplace for the purpose intended by the chemical manufacturer or importer of the product, and the use results in a duration and frequency of exposure which is not greater than the range of exposures that could reasonably be experienced by consumers when used for the purpose intended; (x) Nuisance particulates where the chemical manufacturer or importer can establish that they do not pose any physical or health hazard covered under this section; (xi) Ionizing and nonionizing radiation; and, (xii) Biological hazards.

(c) Definitions. Article means a manufactured item other than a fluid or particle: (I) which is formed to a specific shape or design during manufacture; (ii) which has end use function(s) dependent in whole or in part upon its shape or design during end use; and (iii) which under normal conditions of use does not release more than very small quantities, e.g., minute or trace amounts of a hazardous chemical (as determined under paragraph (d) of this section), and does not pose a physical hazard or health risk to employees. Assistant Secretary means the Assistant Secretary of Labor for Occupational Safety and Health, U.S. Department of Labor, or designee. Chemical means any element, chemical compound or mixture of elements and/or compounds. Chemical manufacturer means an employer with a workplace where chemical(s) are produced for use or distribution. Chemical name means the scientific designation of a chemical in accordance with the nomenclature system developed by the International Union of Pure and Applied Chemistry (IUPAC) or the Chemical Abstracts Service (CAS) rules of nomenclature, or a name which will clearly identify the chemical for the purpose of conducting a hazard evaluation. Combustible liquid means any liquid having a flashpoint at or above 100 degrees F (37.8 degrees C), but below 200 degrees F (93.3 degrees C), except any mixture having components with flashpoints of 200 degrees F (93.3 degrees C), or higher, the total volume of which make up 99 percent or more of the total volume of the mixture. Commercial account means an arrangement whereby a retail distributor sells hazardous chemicals to an employer, generally in large quantities over time and/or at costs that are below the regular retail price. Common name means any designation or identification such as code name, code number, trade name, brand name or generic name used to identify a chemical other than by its chemical name. Compressed gas means: (I) A gas or mixture of gases having, in a container, an absolute pressure exceeding 40 psi at 70 degrees F (21.1 degrees C); or (ii) A gas or mixture of gases having, in a container, an absolute pressure exceeding 104 psi at 130 degrees F (54.4 degrees C) regardless of the pressure at 70 degrees F (21.1 degrees C); or (iii) A liquid having a vapor pressure exceeding 40 psi at 100 degrees F (37.8 degrees C) as determined by ASTM D-323-72. Container means any bag, barrel, bottle, box, can, cylinder, drum, reaction vessel, storage tank, or the like that contains a hazardous chemical. For purposes of this section, pipes or piping systems, and engines, fuel tanks, or other operating systems in a vehicle, are not considered to be containers. Designated representative means any individual or organization to whom an employee gives written authorization to exercise such employee's rights under this section. A recognized or certified collective bargaining agent shall be treated automatically as a designated representative without regard to written employee authorization. Director means the Director, National Institute for Occupational Safety and Health, U.S. Department of Health and Human Services, or designee. Distributor means a business, other than a chemical manufacturer or importer, which supplies hazardous chemicals to other distributors or to employers. Employee means a worker who may be exposed to hazardous chemicals under normal operating conditions or in foreseeable emergencies. Workers such as office workers or bank tellers who encounter hazardous chemicals only in non-routine, isolated instances are not covered. Employer means a person engaged in a business where chemicals are either used, distributed, or are

Appendix B   Hazard Communication   285

produced for use or distribution, including a contractor or subcontractor. Explosive means a chemical that causes a sudden, almost instantaneous release of pressure, gas, and heat when subjected to sudden shock, pressure, or high temperature. Exposure or exposed means that an employee is subjected in the course of employment to a chemical that is a physical or health hazard, and includes potential (e.g. accidental or possible) exposure. 'Subjected' in terms of health hazards includes any route of entry (e.g. inhalation, ingestion, skin contact or absorption.) Flammable means a chemical that falls into one of the following categories: (I) Aerosol, flammable means an aerosol that, when tested by the method described in 16 CFR 1500.45, yields a flame projection exceeding 18 inches at full valve opening, or a flashback (a flame extending back to the valve) at any degree of valve opening; (ii) Gas, flammable means: (A) A gas that, at ambient temperature and pressure, forms a flammable mixture with air at a concentration of thirteen (13) percent by volume or less; or (B) A gas that, at ambient temperature and pressure, forms a range of flammable mixtures with air wider than twelve (12) percent by volume, regardless of the lower limit; (iii) Liquid, flammable means any liquid having a flashpoint below 100 degrees F (37.8 degrees C), except any mixture having components with flashpoints of 100 degrees F (37.8 degrees C) or higher, the total of which make up 99 percent or more of the total volume of the mixture. (iv) Solid, flammable means a solid, other than a blasting agent or explosive as defined in Sec. 1910.109(a), that is liable to cause fire through friction, absorption of moisture, spontaneous chemical change, or retained heat from manufacturing or processing, or which can be ignited readily and when ignited burns so vigorously and persistently as to create a serious hazard. A chemical shall be considered to be a flammable solid if, when tested by the method described in 16 CFR 1500.44, it ignites and burns with a self-sustained flame at a rate greater than one-tenth of an inch per second along its major axis. Flashpoint means the minimum temperature at which a liquid gives off a vapor in sufficient concentration to ignite when tested as follows: (I) Tagliabue Closed Tester (See American National Standard Method of Test for Flash Point by Tag Closed Tester, Z11.24-1979 (ASTM D 56-79)) for liquids with a viscosity of less than 45 Saybolt Universal Seconds (SUS) at 100 degrees F (37.8 degrees C), that do not contain suspended solids and do not have a tendency to form a surface film under test; or (ii) Pensky-Martens Closed Tester (see American National Standard Method of Test for Flash Point by Pensky-Martens Closed Tester, Z11.7-1979 (ASTM D 93-79)) for liquids with a viscosity equal to or greater than 45 SUS at 100 degrees F (37.8 degrees C), or that contain suspended solids, or that have a tendency to form a surface film under test; or (iii) Setaflash Closed Tester (see American National Standard Method of Test for Flash Point by Setaflash Closed Tester (ASTM D3278-78)). Organic peroxides, which undergo autoaccelerating thermal decomposition, are excluded from any of the flashpoint determination methods specified above. Foreseeable emergency means any potential occurrence such as, but not limited to, equipment failure, rupture of containers, or failure of control equipment which could result in an uncontrolled release of a hazardous chemical into the workplace. Hazardous chemical means any chemical which is a physical hazard or a health hazard. Hazard warning means any words, pictures, symbols, or combination thereof appearing on a label or other appropriate form of warning which convey the specific physical and health hazard(s), including target organ effects, of the chemical(s) in the container(s). (See the definitions for 'physical hazard' and 'health hazard' to determine the hazards which must be covered.) Health hazard means a chemical for which there is statistically significant evidence based on at least one study conducted in accordance with established scientific principles that acute or chronic health effects may occur in exposed employees. The term 'health hazard' includes chemicals which are carcinogens, toxic or highly toxic agents, reproductive toxins, irritants, corrosives, sensitizers, hepatotoxins, nephrotoxins, neurotoxins, agents which act on the hematopoietic system, and agents which damage the lungs, skin, eyes, or mucous membranes. Appendix A provides further definitions and explanations of the scope of health hazards covered by this section, and Appendix B describes the criteria to be used to determine whether or not a chemical is to be considered hazardous for purposes of this standard. Identity means any chemical or common name which is indicated on the material safety data sheet (MSDS) for the chemical. The identity used shall permit cross-references to be made among the required list of hazardous chemicals, the label and the MSDS. Immediate use means that the hazardous chemical will be under the control of and used only by the person who transfers it from a labeled container and only within the work shift in which it is transferred. Importer means the first business with employees within the Customs Territory of the United States which receives hazardous chemicals produced in other countries for the purpose of supplying them to distributors or employers within the United States. Label means any written, printed, or graphic material displayed on or affixed to containers of hazardous chemicals. Material safety data sheet (MSDS) means written or printed material concerning a hazardous chemical which is prepared in accordance with paragraph (g) of this section. Mixture means any combination of two or more chemicals if the combination is not, in whole or in part, the result of a chemical reaction. Organic peroxide means an organic compound that contains the bivalent -O-O-structure and which may be considered to be a structural derivative of hydrogen peroxide where one or both of the hydrogen atoms has been replaced by an organic radical. Oxidizer means a chemical other than a blasting agent or explosive as defined in Sec. 1910.109(a), that initiates or promotes combustion in other materials, thereby causing fire either of itself or through the release of oxygen or other gases. Physical hazard means a chemical for which there is scientifically valid evidence that it is a combustible liquid, a compressed gas, explosive, flammable, an organic peroxide, an oxidizer, pyrophoric, unstable (reactive) or water-reactive. Produce means to manufacture, process, formulate, blend, extract, generate, emit, or repackage. Pyrophoric means a chemical that will ignite spontaneously in air at a temperature of 130 degrees F (54.4 degrees C) or below. Responsible party means someone who can provide additional information on the hazardous chemical and appropriate emergency procedures, if necessary. Specific chemical identity means the chemical name, Chemical Abstracts Service (CAS) Registry Number, or any other information that reveals the precise chemical designation of the substance. Trade secret means any confidential formula, pattern, process, device, information or compilation of information that is used in an employer's business, and that gives the employer an opportunity to obtain an advantage over competitors who do not know or use it. Appendix D sets out the criteria to be used in evaluating trade secrets. Unstable (reactive) means a chemical which in the pure state, or as produced or transported, will vigorously polymerize, decompose, condense, or will become self-reactive under conditions of shocks, pressure or temperature. Use means to package, handle, react, emit, extract, generate as a byproduct, or transfer. Water-reactive means a chemical that reacts with water to release a gas that is either flammable or presents a health hazard. Work area means a room or defined space in a workplace where hazardous chemicals are produced or used, and where employees are present. Workplace means an establishment, job site, or project, at one geographical location containing one or more work areas.

(d) Hazard determination. (1) Chemical manufacturers and importers shall evaluate chemicals produced in their workplaces or imported by them to determine if they are hazardous. Employers are not required to evaluate chemicals unless they choose not to rely on the evaluation performed by the chemical manufacturer or importer for the chemical to satisfy this requirement. (2) Chemical manufacturers, importers or employers evaluating chemicals shall identify and consider the available scientific evidence concerning such hazards. For health hazards, evidence which is statistically significant and which is based on at least one positive study conducted in accordance with established scientific principles is considered to be sufficient to establish a hazardous effect if the results of the study meet the definitions of health hazards in this section. Appendix A shall be consulted for the scope of health hazards covered, and Appendix B shall be consulted for the criteria to be followed with respect to the completeness of the evaluation, and the data to be reported. (3) The chemical manufacturer, importer or employer evaluating chemicals shall treat the following sources as establishing that the chemicals listed in them are hazardous: (I) 29 CFR part 1910, subpart Z, Toxic and Hazardous Substances, Occupational Safety and Health Administration (OSHA); or, (ii) Threshold Limit Values for Chemical Substances and Physical Agents in the Work Environment, American Conference of Governmental Industrial Hygienists (ACGIH) (latest edition). The chemical manufacturer, importer, or employer is still responsible for evaluating the hazards associated with the chemicals in these source lists in accordance with the requirements of this standard. (4) Chemical manufacturers, importers and employers evaluating chemicals shall treat the following sources as establishing that a chemical is a carcinogen or potential carcinogen for hazard communication purposes: (I) National Toxicology Program (NTP), Annual Report on Carcinogens (latest edition); (ii) International Agency for Research on Cancer (IARC) Monographs (latest editions); or (iii) 29 CFR part 1910, subpart Z, Toxic and Hazardous Substances, Occupational Safety and Health Administration. Note: The Registry of Toxic Effects of Chemical Substances published by the National Institute for Occupational Safety and Health indicates whether a chemical has been found by NTP or IARC to be a potential carcinogen. (5) The chemical manufacturer, importer or employer shall determine the hazards of mixtures of chemicals as follows: (I) If a mixture has been tested as a whole to determine its hazards, the results of such testing shall be used to determine whether the mixture is hazardous;

(ii) If a mixture has not been tested as a whole to determine whether the mixture is a health hazard, the mixture shall be assumed to present the same health hazards as do the components which comprise one percent (by weight or volume) or greater of the mixture, except that the mixture shall be assumed to present a carcinogenic hazard if it contains a component in concentrations of 0.1 percent or greater which is considered to be a carcinogen under paragraph (d)(4) of this section; (iii) If a mixture has not been tested as a whole to determine whether the mixture is a physical hazard, the chemical manufacturer, importer, or employer may use whatever scientifically valid data is available to evaluate the physical hazard potential of the mixture; and, (iv) If the chemical manufacturer, importer, or employer has evidence to indicate that a component present in the mixture in concentrations of less than one percent (or in the case of carcinogens, less than 0.1 percent) could be released in concentrations which would exceed an established OSHA permissible exposure limit or ACGIH Threshold Limit Value, or could present a health risk to employees in those concentrations, the mixture shall be assumed to present the same hazard. (6) Chemical manufacturers, importers, or employers evaluating chemicals shall describe in writing the procedures they use to determine the hazards of the chemical they evaluate. The written procedures are to be made available, upon request, to employees, their designated representatives, the Assistant Secretary and the Director. The written description may be incorporated into the written hazard communication program required under paragraph (e) of this section.

(e) Written hazard communication program. (1) Employers shall develop, implement, and maintain at each workplace, a written hazard communication program which at least describes how the criteria specified in paragraphs (f), (g), and (h) of this section for labels and other forms of warning, material safety data sheets, and employee information and training will be met, and which also includes the following: (I) A list of the hazardous chemicals known to be present using an identity that is referenced on the appropriate material safety data sheet (the list may be compiled for the workplace as a whole or for individual work areas); and, (ii) The methods the employer will use to inform employees of the hazards of non-routine tasks (for example, the cleaning of reactor vessels), and the hazards associated with chemicals contained in unlabeled pipes in their work areas. (2) Multi-employer workplaces. Employers who produce, use, or store hazardous chemicals at a workplace in such a way that the employees of other employer(s) may be exposed (for example, employees of a construction contractor working on-site) shall additionally ensure that the hazard communication programs developed and implemented under this paragraph (e) include the following: (I) The methods the employer will use to provide the other employer(s) on-site access to material safety data sheets for each hazardous chemical the other employer(s)' employees may be exposed to while working; (ii) The methods the employer will use to inform the other employer(s) of any precautionary measures that need to be taken to protect employees during the workplace's normal operating conditions and in foreseeable emergencies; and, (iii) The methods the employer will use to inform the other employer(s) of the labeling system used in the workplace. (3) The employer may rely on an existing hazard communication program to comply with these requirements, provided that it meets the criteria established in this paragraph (e). (4) The employer shall make the written hazard communication program available, upon request, to employees, their designated representatives, the Assistant Secretary and the Director, in accordance with the requirements of 29 CFR 1910.20 (e). (5) Where employees must travel between workplaces during a work shift, i.e., their work is carried out at more than one geographical location, the written hazard communication program may be kept at the primary workplace facility.

(f) Labels and other forms of warning. (1) The chemical manufacturer, importer, or distributor shall ensure that each container of hazardous chemicals leaving the workplace is labeled, tagged or marked with the following information: (I) Identity of the hazardous chemical(s); (ii) Appropriate hazard warnings; and (iii) Name and address of the chemical manufacturer, importer, or other responsible party. (2)(I) For solid metal (such as a steel beam or a metal casting), solid wood, or plastic items that are not exempted as articles due to their downstream use, or shipments of whole grain, the required label may be transmitted to the customer at the time of the initial shipment, and need not be included with subsequent shipments to the same employer unless the information on the label changes; (ii) The label may be transmitted with the initial shipment itself, or with the material safety data sheet that is to be provided prior to or at the time of the first shipment; and, (iii) This exception to requiring labels on every container of hazardous chemicals is only for the solid material itself, and does not apply to hazardous chemicals used in conjunction with, or known to be present with, the material and to which employees handling the items in transit may be exposed (for example, cutting fluids or pesticides in grains). (3) Chemical manufacturers, importers, or distributors shall ensure that each container of hazardous chemicals leaving the workplace is labeled, tagged, or marked in accordance with this section in a manner which does not conflict with the requirements of the Hazardous Materials Transportation Act (49 U.S.C. 1801 et seq.) and regulations issued under that Act by the Department of Transportation. (4) If the hazardous chemical is regulated by OSHA in a substance-specific health standard, the chemical manufacturer, importer, distributor or employer shall ensure that the labels or other forms of warning used are in accordance with the requirements of that standard. (5) Except as provided in paragraphs (f)(6) and (f)(7) of this section, the employer shall ensure that each container of hazardous chemicals in the workplace is labeled, tagged or marked with the following information: (I) Identity of the hazardous chemical(s) contained therein; and, (ii) Appropriate hazard warnings, or alternatively, words, pictures, symbols, or combination thereof, which provide at least general information regarding the hazards of the chemicals, and which, in conjunction with the other information immediately available to employees under the hazard communication program, will provide employees with the specific information regarding the physical and health hazards of the hazardous chemical. (6) The employer may use signs, placards, process sheets, batch tickets, operating procedures, or other such written materials in lieu of affixing labels to individual stationary process containers, as long as the alternative method identifies the containers to which it is applicable and conveys the information required by paragraph (f)(5) of this section to be on a label. The written materials shall be readily accessible to the employees in their work area throughout each work shift. (7) The employer is not required to label portable containers into which hazardous chemicals are transferred from labeled containers, and which are intended only for the immediate use of the employee who performs the transfer. For purposes of this section, drugs which are dispensed by a pharmacy to a health care provider for direct administration to a patient are exempted from labeling. (8) The employer shall not remove or deface existing labels on incoming containers of hazardous chemicals, unless the container is immediately marked with the required information. (9) The employer shall ensure that labels or other forms of warning are legible, in English, and prominently displayed on the container, or readily available in the work area throughout each work shift. Employers having employees who speak other languages may add the information in their language to the material presented, as long as the information is presented in English as well. (10) The chemical manufacturer, importer, distributor or employer need not affix new labels to comply with this section if existing labels already convey the required information. (11) Chemical manufacturers, importers, distributors, or employers who become newly aware of any significant information regarding the hazards of a chemical shall revise the labels for the chemical within three months of becoming aware of the new information. Labels on containers of hazardous chemicals shipped after that time shall contain the new information. If the chemical is not currently produced or imported, the chemical manufacturer, importers, distributor, or employer shall add the information to the label before the chemical is shipped or introduced into the workplace again.

(g) Material safety data sheets. (1) Chemical manufacturers and importers shall obtain or develop a material safety data sheet for each hazardous chemical they produce or import. Employers shall have a material safety data sheet in the workplace for each hazardous chemical which they use. (2) Each material safety data sheet shall be in English (although the employer may maintain copies in other languages as well), and shall contain at least the following information: (I) The identity used on the label, and, except as provided for in paragraph (I) of this section on trade secrets: (A) If the hazardous chemical is a single substance, its chemical and common name(s); (B) If the hazardous chemical is a mixture which has been tested as a whole to determine its hazards, the chemical and common name(s) of the ingredients which contribute to these known hazards, and the common name(s) of the mixture itself; or, (C) If the hazardous chemical is a mixture which has not been tested as a whole: (1) The chemical and common name(s) of all ingredients which have been determined to be health hazards, and which comprise 1% or greater of the composition, except that chemicals identified as carcinogens under paragraph (d) of this section shall be listed if the concentrations are 0.1% or greater; and, (2) The chemical and common name(s) of all ingredients which have been determined to be health hazards, and which comprise less than 1% (0.1% for carcinogens) of the mixture, if there is evidence that the ingredient(s) could be released from the mixture in concentrations which would exceed an established OSHA permissible exposure limit or ACGIH Threshold Limit Value, or could present a health risk to employees; and, (3) The chemical and common name(s) of all ingredients which have been determined to present a physical hazard when present in the mixture; (ii) Physical and chemical characteristics of the hazardous chemical (such as vapor pressure, flash point); (iii) The physical hazards of the hazardous chemical, including the potential for fire, explosion, and reactivity; (iv) The health hazards of the hazardous chemical, including signs and symptoms of exposure, and any medical conditions which are generally recognized as being aggravated by exposure to the chemical; (v) The primary route(s) of entry; (vi) The OSHA permissible exposure limit, ACGIH Threshold Limit Value, and any other exposure limit used or recommended by the chemical manufacturer, importer, or employer preparing the material safety data sheet, where available; (vii) Whether the hazardous chemical is listed in the National Toxicology Program (NTP) Annual Report on Carcinogens (latest edition) or has been found to be a potential carcinogen in the International Agency for Research on Cancer (IARC) Monographs (latest editions), or by OSHA; (viii) Any generally applicable precautions for safe handling and use which are known to the chemical manufacturer, importer or employer preparing the material safety data sheet, including appropriate hygienic practices, protective measures during repair and maintenance of contaminated equipment, and procedures for clean-up of spills and leaks; (ix) Any generally applicable control measures which are known to the chemical manufacturer, importer or employer preparing the material safety data sheet, such as appropriate engineering controls, work practices, or personal protective equipment; (x) Emergency and first aid procedures; (xi) The date of preparation of the material safety data sheet or the last change to it; and, (xii) The name, address and telephone number of the chemical manufacturer, importer, employer or other responsible party preparing or distributing the material safety data sheet, who can provide additional information on the hazardous chemical and appropriate emergency procedures, if necessary. (3) If no relevant information is found for any given category on the material safety data sheet, the chemical manufacturer, importer or employer preparing the material safety data sheet shall mark it to indicate that no applicable information was found. (4) Where complex mixtures have similar hazards and contents (i.e. the chemical ingredients are essentially the same, but the specific composition varies from mixture to mixture), the chemical manufacturer, importer or employer may prepare one material safety data sheet to apply to all of these similar mixtures. (5) The chemical manufacturer, importer or employer preparing the material safety data sheet shall ensure that the information recorded accurately reflects the scientific evidence used in making the hazard determination. If the chemical manufacturer, importer or employer preparing the material safety data sheet becomes newly aware of any significant information regarding the hazards of a chemical, or ways to protect against the hazards, this new information shall be added to the material safety data sheet within three months. If the chemical is not currently being produced or imported the chemical manufacturer or importer shall add the information to the material safety data sheet before the chemical is introduced into the workplace again. (6)(I) Chemical manufacturers or importers shall ensure that distributors and employers are provided an appropriate material safety data sheet with their initial shipment, and with the first shipment after a material safety data sheet is updated; (ii) The chemical manufacturer or importer shall either provide material safety data sheets with the shipped containers or send them to the distributor or employer prior to or at the time of the shipment; (iii) If the material safety data sheet is not provided with a shipment that has been labeled as a hazardous chemical, the distributor or employer shall obtain one from the chemical manufacturer or importer as soon as possible; and, (iv) The chemical manufacturer or importer shall also provide distributors or employers with a material safety data sheet upon request. (7)(I) Distributors shall ensure that material safety data sheets, and updated information, are provided to other distributors and employers with their initial shipment and with the first shipment after a material safety data sheet is updated; (ii) The distributor shall either provide material safety data sheets with the shipped containers, or send them to the other distributor or employer prior to or at the time of the shipment; (iii) Retail distributors selling hazardous chemicals to employers having a commercial account shall provide a material safety data sheet to such employers upon request, and shall post a sign or otherwise inform them that a material safety data sheet is available; (iv) Wholesale distributors selling hazardous chemicals to employers over-the-counter may also provide material safety data sheets upon the request of the employer at the time of the over-the-counter purchase, and shall post a sign or otherwise inform such employers that a material safety data sheet is available; (v) If an employer without a commercial account purchases a hazardous chemical from a retail distributor not required to have material safety data sheets on file (i.e., the retail distributor does not have commercial accounts and does not use the materials), the retail distributor shall provide the employer, upon request, with the name, address, and telephone number of the chemical manufacturer, importer, or distributor from which a material safety data sheet can be obtained; (vi) Wholesale distributors shall also provide material safety data sheets to employers or other distributors upon request; and, (vii) Chemical manufacturers, importers, and distributors need not provide material safety data sheets to retail distributors that have informed them that the retail distributor does not sell the product to commercial accounts or open the sealed container to use it in their own workplaces. (8) The employer shall maintain in the workplace copies of the required material safety data sheets for each hazardous chemical, and shall ensure that they are readily accessible during each work shift to employees when they are in their work area(s). (Electronic access, microfiche, and other alternatives to maintaining paper copies of the material safety data sheets are permitted as long as no barriers to immediate employee access in each workplace are created by such options.) (9) Where employees must travel between workplaces during a work shift, i.e., their work is carried out at more than one geographical location, the material safety data sheets may be kept at the primary workplace facility. In this situation, the employer shall ensure that employees can immediately obtain the required information in an emergency. (10) Material safety data sheets may be kept in any form, including operating procedures, and may be designed to cover groups of hazardous chemicals in a work area where it may be more appropriate to address the hazards of a process rather than individual hazardous chemicals. However, the employer shall ensure that in all cases the required information is provided for each hazardous chemical, and is readily accessible during each work shift to employees when they are in their work area(s). (11) Material safety data sheets shall also be made readily available, upon request, to designated representatives and to the Assistant Secretary, in accordance with the requirements of 29 CFR 1910.20(e). The Director shall also be given access to material safety data sheets in the same manner.

(h) Employee information and training. (1) Employers shall provide employees with effective information and training on hazardous chemicals in their work area at the time of their initial assignment, and whenever a new physical or health hazard the employees have not previously been trained about is introduced into their work area. Information and training may be designed to cover categories of hazards (e.g., flammability, carcinogenicity) or specific chemicals. Chemical-specific information must always be available through labels and material safety data sheets. (2) Information. Employees shall be informed of: (I) The requirements of this section; (ii) Any operations in their work area where hazardous chemicals are present; and, (iii) The location and availability of the written hazard communication program, including the required list(s) of hazardous chemicals, and material safety data sheets required by this section. (3) Training. Employee training shall include at least: (I) Methods and observations that may be used to detect the presence or release of a hazardous chemical in the work area (such as monitoring conducted by the employer, continuous monitoring devices, visual appearance or odor of hazardous chemicals when being released, etc.); (ii) The physical and health hazards of the chemicals in the work area; (iii) The measures employees can take to protect themselves from these hazards, including specific procedures the employer has implemented to protect employees from exposure to hazardous chemicals, such as appropriate work practices, emergency procedures, and personal protective equipment to be used; and, (iv) The details of the hazard communication program developed by the employer, including an explanation of the labeling system and the material safety data sheet, and how employees can obtain and use the appropriate hazard information.

(i) Trade secrets. (1) The chemical manufacturer, importer, or employer may withhold the specific chemical identity, including the chemical name and other specific identification of a hazardous chemical, from the material safety data sheet, provided that: (I) The claim that the information withheld is a trade secret can be supported; (ii) Information contained in the material safety data sheet concerning the properties and effects of the hazardous chemical is disclosed; (iii) The material safety data sheet indicates that the specific chemical identity is being withheld as a trade secret; and, (iv) The specific chemical identity is made available to health professionals, employees, and designated representatives in accordance with the applicable provisions of this paragraph. (2) Where a treating physician or nurse determines that a medical emergency exists and the specific chemical identity of a hazardous chemical is necessary for emergency or first-aid treatment, the chemical manufacturer, importer, or employer shall immediately disclose the specific chemical identity of a trade secret chemical to that treating physician or nurse, regardless of the existence of a written statement of need or a confidentiality agreement. The chemical manufacturer, importer, or employer may require a written statement of need and confidentiality agreement, in accordance with the provisions of paragraphs (I) (3) and (4) of this section, as soon as circumstances permit. (3) In non-emergency situations, a chemical manufacturer, importer, or employer shall, upon request, disclose a specific chemical identity, otherwise permitted to be withheld under paragraph (I)(1) of this section, to a health professional (i.e. physician, industrial hygienist, toxicologist, epidemiologist, or occupational health nurse) providing medical or other occupational health services to exposed employee(s), and to employees or designated representatives, if: (I) The request is in writing; (ii) The request describes with reasonable detail one or more of the following occupational health needs for the information: (A) To assess the hazards of the chemicals to which employees will be exposed; (B) To conduct or assess sampling of the workplace atmosphere to determine employee exposure levels; (C) To conduct pre-assignment or periodic medical surveillance of exposed employees; (D) To provide medical treatment to exposed employees; (E) To select or assess appropriate personal protective equipment for exposed employees; (F) To design or assess engineering controls or other protective measures for exposed employees; and, (G) To conduct studies to determine the health effects of exposure. (iii) The request explains in detail why the disclosure of the specific chemical identity is essential and that, in lieu thereof, the disclosure of the following information to the health professional, employee, or designated representative, would not satisfy the purposes described in paragraph (I)(3)(ii) of this section: (A) The properties and effects of the chemical; (B) Measures for controlling workers' exposure to the chemical; (C) Methods of monitoring and analyzing worker exposure to the chemical; and, (D) Methods of diagnosing and treating harmful exposures to the chemical; (iv) The request includes a description of the procedures to be used to maintain the confidentiality of the disclosed information; and, (v) The health professional, and the employer or contractor of the services of the health professional (i.e. downstream employer, labor organization, or individual employee), employee, or designated representative, agree in a written confidentiality agreement that the health professional, employee, or designated representative, will not use the trade secret information for any purpose other than the health need(s) asserted and agree not to release the information under any circumstances other than to OSHA, as provided in paragraph (I)(6) of this section, except as authorized by the terms of the agreement or by the chemical manufacturer, importer, or employer. (4) The confidentiality agreement authorized by paragraph (I)(3)(iv) of this section: (I) May restrict the use of the information to the health purposes indicated in the written statement of need; (ii) May provide for appropriate legal remedies in the event of a breach of the agreement, including stipulation of a reasonable pre-estimate of likely damages; and, (iii) May not include requirements for the posting of a penalty bond. (5) Nothing in this standard is meant to preclude the parties from pursuing non-contractual remedies to the extent permitted by law. (6) If the health professional, employee, or designated representative receiving the trade secret information decides that there is a need to disclose it to OSHA, the chemical manufacturer, importer, or employer who provided the information shall be informed by the health professional, employee, or designated representative prior to, or at the same time as, such disclosure. (7) If the chemical manufacturer, importer, or employer denies a written request for disclosure of a specific chemical identity, the denial must: (I) Be provided to the health professional, employee, or designated representative, within thirty days of the request; (ii) Be in writing; (iii) Include evidence to support the claim that the specific chemical identity is a trade secret; (iv) State the specific reasons why the request is being denied; and, (v) Explain in detail how alternative information may satisfy the specific medical or occupational health need without revealing the specific chemical identity. (8) The health professional, employee, or designated representative whose request for information is denied under paragraph (I)(3) of this section may refer the request and the written denial of the request to OSHA for consideration. (9) When a health professional, employee, or designated representative refers the denial to OSHA under paragraph (I)(8) of this section, OSHA shall consider the evidence to determine if: (I) The chemical manufacturer, importer, or employer has supported the claim that the specific chemical identity is a trade secret; (ii) The health professional, employee, or designated representative has supported the claim that there is a medical or occupational health need for the information; and, (iii) The health professional, employee or designated representative has demonstrated adequate means to protect the confidentiality. (10)(I) If OSHA determines that the specific chemical identity requested under paragraph (I)(3) of this section is not a bona fide trade secret, or that it is a trade secret, but the requesting health professional, employee, or designated representative has a legitimate medical or occupational health need for the information, has executed a written confidentiality agreement, and has shown adequate means to protect the confidentiality of the information, the chemical manufacturer, importer, or employer will be subject to citation by OSHA. (ii) If a chemical manufacturer, importer, or employer demonstrates to OSHA that the execution of a confidentiality agreement would not provide sufficient protection against the potential harm from the unauthorized disclosure of a trade secret specific chemical identity, the Assistant Secretary may issue such orders or impose such additional limitations or conditions upon the disclosure of the requested chemical information as may be appropriate to assure that the occupational health services are provided without an undue risk of harm to the chemical manufacturer, importer, or employer. (11) If a citation for a failure to release specific chemical identity information is contested by the chemical manufacturer, importer, or employer, the matter will be adjudicated before the Occupational Safety and Health Review Commission in accordance with the Act's enforcement scheme and the applicable Commission rules of procedure. In accordance with the Commission rules, when a chemical manufacturer, importer, or employer continues to withhold the information during the contest, the Administrative Law Judge may review the citation and supporting documentation in camera or issue appropriate orders to protect the confidentiality of such matters. (12) Notwithstanding the existence of a trade secret claim, a chemical manufacturer, importer, or employer shall, upon request, disclose to the Assistant Secretary any information which this section requires the chemical manufacturer, importer, or employer to make available. Where there is a trade secret claim, such claim shall be made no later than at the time the information is provided to the Assistant Secretary so that suitable determinations of trade secret status can be made and the necessary protections can be implemented. (13) Nothing in this paragraph shall be construed as requiring the disclosure under any circumstances of process or percentage of mixture information which is a trade secret.

(j) Effective dates. Chemical manufacturers, importers, distributors, and employers shall be in compliance with all provisions of this section by March 11, 1994. Note: The effective date of the clarification that the exemption of wood and wood products from the Hazard Communication standard in paragraph (b)(6)(iv) only applies to wood and wood products including lumber which will not be processed, where the manufacturer or importer can establish that the only hazard they pose to employees is the potential for flammability or combustibility, and that the exemption does not apply to wood or wood products which have been treated with a hazardous chemical covered by this standard, and wood which may be subsequently sawed or cut generating dust has been stayed from March 11, 1994 to August 11, 1994.

APPENDIX C

BLOODBORNE PATHOGENS STANDARD
29 CFR 1910.1030

(a) Scope and Application. This section applies to all occupational exposure to blood or other potentially infectious materials as defined by paragraph (b) of this section.

(b) Definitions. For purposes of this section, the following shall apply: Assistant Secretary means the Assistant Secretary of Labor for Occupational Safety and Health, or designated representative. Blood means human blood, human blood components, and products made from human blood. Bloodborne Pathogens means pathogenic microorganisms that are present in human blood and can cause disease in humans. These pathogens include, but are not limited to, hepatitis B virus (HBV) and human immunodeficiency virus (HIV). Clinical Laboratory means a workplace where diagnostic or other screening procedures are performed on blood or other potentially infectious materials. Contaminated means the presence or the reasonably anticipated presence of blood or other potentially infectious materials on an item or surface. Contaminated Laundry means laundry which has been soiled with blood or other potentially infectious materials or may contain sharps. Contaminated Sharps means any contaminated object that can penetrate the skin including, but not limited to, needles, scalpels, broken glass, broken capillary tubes, and exposed ends of dental wires. Decontamination means the use of physical or chemical means to remove, inactivate, or destroy bloodborne pathogens on a surface or item to the point where they are no longer capable of transmitting infectious particles and the surface or item is rendered safe for handling, use, or disposal. Director means the Director of the National Institute for Occupational Safety and Health, U.S. Department of Health and Human Services, or designated representative. Engineering Controls means controls (e.g., sharps disposal containers, self-sheathing needles) that isolate or remove the bloodborne pathogens hazard from the workplace. Exposure Incident means a specific eye, mouth, other mucous membrane, non-intact skin, or parenteral contact with blood or other potentially infectious materials that results from the performance of an employee's duties. Handwashing Facilities means a facility providing an adequate supply of running potable water, soap and single use towels or hot air drying machines. Licensed Healthcare Professional is a person whose legally permitted scope of practice allows him or her to independently perform the activities required by paragraph (f) Hepatitis B Vaccination and Post-exposure Evaluation and Follow-up. HBV means hepatitis B virus. HIV means human immunodeficiency virus. Occupational Exposure means reasonably anticipated skin, eye, mucous membrane, or parenteral contact with blood or other potentially infectious materials that may result from the performance of an employee's duties. Other Potentially Infectious Materials means (1) The following human body fluids: semen, vaginal secretions, cerebrospinal fluid, synovial fluid, pleural fluid, pericardial fluid, peritoneal fluid, amniotic fluid, saliva in dental procedures, any body fluid that is visibly contaminated with blood, and all body fluids in situations where it is difficult or impossible to differentiate between body fluids; (2) Any unfixed tissue or organ (other than intact skin) from a human (living or dead); and (3) HIV-containing cell or tissue cultures, organ cultures, and HIV- or HBV-containing culture medium or other solutions; and blood, organs, or other tissues from experimental animals infected with HIV or HBV. Parenteral means piercing mucous membranes or the skin barrier through such events as needlesticks, human bites, cuts, and abrasions. Personal Protective Equipment is specialized clothing or equipment worn by an employee for protection against a hazard. General work clothes (e.g., uniforms, pants, shirts or blouses) not intended to function as protection against a hazard are not considered to be personal protective equipment. Production Facility means a facility engaged in industrial-scale, large-volume or high concentration production of HIV or HBV. Regulated Waste means liquid or semi-liquid blood or other potentially infectious materials; contaminated items that would release blood or other potentially infectious materials in a liquid or semi-liquid state if compressed; items that are caked with dried blood or other potentially infectious materials and are capable of releasing these materials during handling; contaminated sharps; and pathological and microbiological wastes containing blood or other potentially infectious materials. Research Laboratory means a laboratory producing or using research-laboratory-scale amounts of HIV or HBV. Research laboratories may produce high concentrations of HIV or HBV but not in the volume found in production facilities. Source Individual means any individual, living or dead, whose blood or other potentially infectious materials may be a source of occupational exposure to the employee. Examples include, but are not limited to, hospital and clinic patients; clients in institutions for the developmentally disabled; trauma victims; clients of drug and alcohol treatment facilities; residents of hospices and nursing homes; human remains; and individuals who donate or sell blood or blood components. Sterilize means the use of a physical or chemical procedure to destroy all microbial life including highly resistant bacterial endospores. Universal Precautions is an approach to infection control. According to the concept of Universal Precautions, all human blood and certain human body fluids are treated as if known to be infectious for HIV, HBV, and other bloodborne pathogens. Work Practice Controls means controls that reduce the likelihood of exposure by altering the manner in which a task is performed (e.g., prohibiting recapping of needles by a two-handed technique).

(c) **Exposure control** - (1) Exposure Control Plan. (I) Each employer having an employee(s) with occupational exposure as defined by paragraph (b) of this section shall establish a written Exposure Control Plan designed to eliminate or minimize employee exposure. (ii) The Exposure Control Plan shall contain at least the following elements: (A) The exposure determination required by paragraph(c)(2), (B) The schedule and method of implementation for paragraphs (d) Methods of Compliance, (e) HIV and HBV Research Laboratories and Production Facilities, (f) Hepatitis B Vaccination and Post-Exposure Evaluation and Follow-up, (g) Communication of Hazards to Employees, and (h)

Recordkeeping, of this standard, and (C) The procedure for the evaluation of circumstances surrounding exposure incidents as required by paragraph (f)(3)(I) of this standard. (iii) Each employer shall ensure that a copy of the Exposure Control Plan is accessible to employees in accordance with 29 CFR 1910.20(e). (iv) The Exposure Control Plan shall be reviewed and updated at least annually and whenever necessary to reflect new or modified tasks and procedures which affect occupational exposure and to reflect new or revised employee positions with occupational exposure. (v) The Exposure Control Plan shall be made available to the Assistant Secretary and the Director upon request for examination and copying. (2) Exposure determination. (I) Each employer who has an employee(s) with occupational exposure as defined by paragraph (b) of this section shall prepare an exposure determination. This exposure determination shall contain the following: (A) A list of all job classifications in which all employees in those job classifications have occupational exposure; (B) A list of job classifications in which some employees have occupational exposure, and (C) A list of all tasks and procedures or groups of closely related task and procedures in which occupational exposure occurs and that are performed by employees in job classifications listed in accordance with the provisions of paragraph (c)(2)(I)(B) of this standard. (ii) This exposure determination shall be made without regard to the use of personal protective equipment.

(d) Methods of compliance - (1) General - Universal precautions shall be observed to prevent contact with blood or other potentially infectious materials. Under circumstances in which differentiation between body fluid types is difficult or impossible, all body fluids shall be considered potentially infectious materials.
(2) Engineering and work practice controls. (I) Engineering and work practice controls shall be used to eliminate or minimize employee exposure. Where occupational exposure remains after institution of these controls, personal protective equipment shall also be used. (ii) Engineering controls shall be examined and maintained or replaced on a regular schedule to ensure their effectiveness. (iii) Employers shall provide handwashing facilities which are readily accessible to employees. (iv) When provision of handwashing facilities is not feasible, the employer shall provide either an appropriate antiseptic hand cleanser in conjunction with clean cloth/paper towels or antiseptic towelettes. When antiseptic hand cleansers or towelettes are used, hands shall be washed with soap and running water as soon as feasible. (v) Employers shall ensure that employees wash their hands immediately or as soon as feasible after removal of gloves or other personal protective equipment. (vi) Employers shall ensure that employees wash hands and any other skin with soap and water, or flush mucous membranes with water immediately or as soon as feasible following contact of such body areas with blood or other potentially infectious materials. (vii) Contaminated needles and other contaminated sharps shall not be bent, recapped, or removed except as noted in paragraphs (d)(2)(vii)(A) and (d)(2)(vii)(B) below. Shearing or breaking of contaminated needles is prohibited. (A) Contaminated needles and other contaminated sharps shall not be bent, recapped or removed unless the employer can demonstrate that no alternative is feasible or that such action is required by a specific medical or dental procedure. (B) Such bending, recapping

or needle removal must be accomplished through the use of a mechanical device or a one-handed technique. (viii) Immediately or as soon as possible after use, contaminated reusable sharps shall be placed in appropriate containers until properly reprocessed. These containers shall be: (A) Puncture resistant; (B) Labeled or color-coded in accordance with this standard; (C) Leakproof on the sides and bottom; and (D) In accordance with the requirements set forth in paragraph (d)(4)(ii)(E) for reusable sharps. (ix) Eating, drinking, smoking, applying cosmetics or lip balm, and handling contact lenses are prohibited in work areas where there is a reasonable likelihood of occupational exposure. (x) Food and drink shall not be kept in refrigerators, freezers, shelves, cabinets or on countertops or benchtops where blood or other potentially infectious materials are present. (xi) All procedures involving blood or other potentially infectious materials shall be performed in such a manner as to minimize splashing, spraying, spattering, and generation of droplets of these substances. (xii) Mouth pipetting/suctioning of blood or other potentially infectious materials is prohibited. (xiii) Specimens of blood or other potentially infectious materials shall be placed in a container which prevents leakage during collection, handling, processing, storage, transport, or shipping. (A) The container for storage, transport, or shipping shall be labeled or color-coded according to paragraph (g)(1)(I) and closed prior to being stored, transported, or shipped. When a facility utilizes Universal Precautions in the handling of all specimens, the labeling/color-coding of specimens is not necessary provided containers are recognizable as containing specimens. This exemption only applies while such specimens/containers remain within the facility. Labeling or color-coding in accordance with paragraph (g)(1)(I) is required when such specimens/containers leave the facility. (B) If outside contamination of the primary container occurs, the primary container shall be placed within a second container which prevents leakage during handling, processing, storage, transport, or shipping and is labeled or color-coded according to the requirements of this standard. (C) If the specimen could puncture the primary container, the primary container shall be placed within a secondary container which is puncture-resistant in addition to the above characteristics.

(xiv) Equipment which may become contaminated with blood or other potentially infectious materials shall be examined prior to servicing or shipping and shall be decontaminated as necessary, unless the employer can demonstrate that decontamination of such equipment or portions of such equipment is not feasible. (A) A readily observable label in accordance with paragraph (g)(1)(I)(H) shall be attached to the equipment stating which portions remain contaminated. (B) The employer shall ensure that this information is conveyed to all affected employees, the servicing representative, and/or the manufacturer, as appropriate, prior to handling, servicing, or shipping so that appropriate precautions will be taken.

(3) Personal protective equipment - (I) Provision. When there is occupational exposure, the employer shall provide, at no cost to the employee, appropriate personal protective equipment such as, but not limited to, gloves, gowns, laboratory coats, face shields or masks and eye protection, and mouthpieces, resuscitation bags, pocket masks, or other ventilation devices. Personal protective equipment will be considered 'appropriate' only if it does not permit blood or other potentially infectious materials to pass through to or

reach the employee's work clothes, street clothes, undergarments, skin, eyes, mouth, or other mucous membranes under normal conditions of use and for the duration of time which the protective equipment will be used. (ii) Use. The employer shall ensure that the employee uses appropriate personal protective equipment unless the employer shows that the employee temporarily and briefly declined to use personal protective equipment when, under rare and extraordinary circumstances, it was the employee's professional judgment that in the specific instance its use would have prevented the delivery of health care or public safety services or would have posed an increased hazard to the safety of the worker or co-worker. When the employee makes this judgement, the circumstances shall be investigated and documented in order to determine whether changes can be instituted to prevent such occurrences in the future. (iii) Accessibility. The employer shall ensure that appropriate personal protective equipment in the appropriate sizes is readily accessible at the worksite or is issued to employees. Hypoallergenic gloves, glove liners, powderless gloves, or other similar alternatives shall be readily accessible to those employees who are allergic to the gloves normally provided. (iv) Cleaning, Laundering, and Disposal. The employer shall clean, launder, and dispose of personal protective equipment required by paragraphs (d) and (e) of this standard, at no cost to the employee. (v) Repair and Replacement. The employer shall repair or replace personal protective equipment as needed to maintain its effectiveness, at no cost to the employee. (vi) If a garment(s) is penetrated by blood or other potentially infectious materials, the garment(s) shall be removed immediately or as soon as feasible. (vii) All personal protective equipment shall be removed prior to leaving the work area. (viii) When personal protective equipment is removed it shall be placed in an appropriately designated area or container for storage, washing, decontamination or disposal. (ix) Gloves. Gloves shall be worn when it can be reasonably anticipated that the employee may have hand contact with blood, other potentially infectious materials, mucous membranes, and non-intact skin; when performing vascular access procedures except as specified in paragraph (d)(3)(ix)(D); and when handling or touching contaminated items or surfaces. (A) Disposable (single use) gloves such as surgical or examination gloves, shall be replaced as soon as practical when contaminated or as soon as feasible if they are torn, punctured, or when their ability to function as a barrier is compromised. (B) Disposable (single use) gloves shall not be washed or decontaminated for re-use. (C) Utility gloves may be decontaminated for re-use if the integrity of the glove is not compromised. However, they must be discarded if they are cracked, peeling, torn, punctured, or exhibit other signs of deterioration or when their ability to function as a barrier is compromised. (D) If an employer in a volunteer blood donation center judges that routine gloving for all phlebotomies is not necessary then the employer shall: (1) Periodically reevaluate this policy; (2) Make gloves available to all employees who wish to use them for phlebotomy; (3) Not discourage the use of gloves for phlebotomy; and (4) Require that gloves be used for phlebotomy in the following circumstances: (I) When the employee has cuts, scratches, or other breaks in his or her skin; (ii) When the employee judges that hand contamination with blood may occur, for example, when performing phlebotomy on an uncooperative source individual; and (iii) When the employee is receiving training in phlebotomy. (x) Masks, Eye Protection, and Face Shields. Masks in combination with eye protection devices, such as goggles or glasses with solid side shields, or chin-length face shields, shall be worn whenever splashes, spray, spatter, or droplets of blood or other potentially infectious materials may be generated and eye, nose, or mouth contamination can be reasonably anticipated. (xi) Gowns, Aprons, and Other Protective Body Clothing. Appropriate protective clothing such as, but not limited to, gowns, aprons, lab coats, clinic jackets, or similar outer garments shall be worn in occupational exposure situations. The type and characteristics will depend upon the task and degree of exposure anticipated. (xii) Surgical caps or hoods and/or shoe covers or boots shall be worn in instances when gross contamination can reasonably be anticipated (e.g., autopsies, orthopaedic surgery).

(4) Housekeeping. (I) General. Employers shall ensure that the worksite is maintained in a clean and sanitary condition. The employer shall determine and implement an appropriate written schedule for cleaning and method of decontamination based upon the location within the facility, type of surface to be cleaned, type of soil present, and tasks or procedures being performed in the area. (ii) All equipment and environmental and working surfaces shall be cleaned and decontaminated after contact with blood or other potentially infectious materials. (A) Contaminated work surfaces shall be decontaminated with an appropriate disinfectant after completion of procedures; immediately or as soon as feasible when surfaces are overtly contaminated or after any spill of blood or other potentially infectious materials; and at the end of the work shift if the surface may have become contaminated since the last cleaning. (B) Protective coverings, such as plastic wrap, aluminum foil, or imperviously-backed absorbent paper used to cover equipment and environmental surfaces, shall be removed and replaced as soon as feasible when they become overtly contaminated or at the end of the work shift if they may have become contaminated during the shift. (C) All bins, pails, cans, and similar receptacles intended for reuse which have a reasonable likelihood for becoming contaminated with blood or other potentially infectious materials shall be inspected and decontaminated on a regularly scheduled basis and cleaned and decontaminated immediately or as soon as feasible upon visible contamination. (D) Broken glassware which may be contaminated shall not be picked up directly with the hands. It shall be cleaned up using mechanical means, such as a brush and dust pan, tongs, or forceps. (E) Reusable sharps that are contaminated with blood or other potentially infectious materials shall not be stored or processed in a manner that requires employees to reach by hand into the containers where these sharps have been placed. (iii) Regulated Waste. (A) Contaminated Sharps Discarding and Containment. (1) Contaminated sharps shall be discarded immediately or as soon as feasible in containers that are: (I) Closable; (ii) Puncture resistant; (iii) Leakproof on sides and bottom; and (iv) Labeled or color-coded in accordance with paragraph (g)(1)(I) of this standard. (2) During use, containers for contaminated sharps shall be: (I) Easily accessible to personnel and located as close as is feasible to the immediate area where sharps are used or can be reasonably anticipated to be found (e.g., laundries); (ii) Maintained upright throughout use; and (iii) Replaced routinely and not be allowed to overfill. (3) When moving containers of contaminated sharps from the area

of use, the containers shall be: (I) Closed immediately prior to removal or replacement to prevent spillage or protrusion of contents during handling, storage, transport, or shipping; (ii) Placed in a secondary container if leakage is possible. The second container shall be: (A) Closable; (B) Constructed to contain all contents and prevent leakage during handling, storage, transport, or shipping; and (C) Labeled or color-coded according to paragraph (g)(1)(I) of this standard. (4) Reusable containers shall not be opened, emptied, or cleaned manually or in any other manner which would expose employees to the risk of percutaneous injury. (B) Other Regulated Waste Containment. (1) Regulated waste shall be placed in containers which are: (I) Closable; (ii) Constructed to contain all contents and prevent leakage of fluids during handling, storage, transport or shipping; (iii) Labeled or color-coded in accordance with paragraph (g)(1)(I) this standard; and (iv) Closed prior to removal to prevent spillage or protrusion of contents during handling, storage, transport, or shipping. (2) If outside contamination of the regulated waste container occurs, it shall be placed in a second container. The second container shall be: (I) Closable; (ii) Constructed to contain all contents and prevent leakage of fluids during handling, storage, transport or shipping; (iii) Labeled or color-coded in accordance with paragraph (g)(1)(I) of this standard; and (iv) Closed prior to removal to prevent spillage or protrusion of contents during handling, storage, transport, or shipping. (C) Disposal of all regulated waste shall be in accordance with applicable regulations of the United States, States and Territories, and political subdivisions of States and Territories. (iv) Laundry. (A) Contaminated laundry shall be handled as little as possible with a minimum of agitation. (1) Contaminated laundry shall be bagged or containerized at the location where it was used and shall not be sorted or rinsed in the location of use. (2) Contaminated laundry shall be placed and transported in bags or containers labeled or color-coded in accordance with paragraph (g)(1)(I) of this standard. When a facility utilizes Universal Precautions in the handling of all soiled laundry, alternative labeling or color-coding is sufficient if it permits all employees to recognize the containers as requiring compliance with Universal Precautions. (3) Whenever contaminated laundry is wet and presents a reasonable likelihood of soak-through of or leakage from the bag or container, the laundry shall be placed and transported in bags or containers which prevent soak-through and/or leakage of fluids to the exterior. (B) The employer shall ensure that employees who have contact with contaminated laundry wear protective gloves and other appropriate personal protective equipment. (C) When a facility ships contaminated laundry off-site to a second facility which does not utilize Universal Precautions in the handling of all laundry, the facility generating the contaminated laundry must place such laundry in bags or containers which are labeled or color-coded in accordance with paragraph (g)(1)(I).

(e) HIV and HBV Research Laboratories and Production Facilities.
(1) This paragraph applies to research laboratories and production facilities engaged in the culture, production, concentration, experimentation, and manipulation of HIV and HBV. It does not apply to clinical or diagnostic laboratories engaged solely in the analysis of blood, tissues, or organs. These requirements apply in addition to the other

requirements of the standard. (2) Research laboratories and production facilities shall meet the following criteria: (I) Standard microbiological practices. All regulated waste shall either be incinerated or decontaminated by a method such as autoclaving known to effectively destroy bloodborne pathogens. (ii) Special practices. (A) Laboratory doors shall be kept closed when work involving HIV or HBV is in progress. (B) Contaminated materials that are to be decontaminated at a site away from the work area shall be placed in a durable, leakproof, labeled or color-coded container that is closed before being removed from the work area. (C) Access to the work area shall be limited to authorized persons. Written policies and procedures shall be established whereby only persons who have been advised of the potential biohazard, who meet any specific entry requirements, and who comply with all entry and exit procedures shall be allowed to enter the work areas and animal rooms. (D) When other potentially infectious materials or infected animals are present in the work area or containment module, a hazard warning sign incorporating the universal biohazard symbol shall be posted on all access doors. The hazard warning sign shall comply with paragraph (g)(1)(ii) of this standard. (E) All activities involving other potentially infectious materials shall be conducted in biological safety cabinets or other physical-containment devices within the containment module. No work with these other potentially infectious materials shall be conducted on the open bench. (F) Laboratory coats, gowns, smocks, uniforms, or other appropriate protective clothing shall be used in the work area and animal rooms. Protective clothing shall not be worn outside of the work area and shall be decontaminated before being laundered. (G) Special care shall be taken to avoid skin contact with other potentially infectious materials. Gloves shall be worn when handling infected animals and when making hand contact with other potentially infectious materials is unavoidable. (H) Before disposal all waste from work areas and from animal rooms shall either be incinerated or decontaminated by a method such as autoclaving known to effectively destroy bloodborne pathogens. (I) Vacuum lines shall be protected with liquid disinfectant traps and high-efficiency particulate air (HEPA) filters or filters of equivalent or superior efficiency and which are checked routinely and maintained or replaced as necessary. (J) Hypodermic needles and syringes shall be used only for parenteral injection and aspiration of fluids from laboratory animals and diaphragm bottles. Only needle-locking syringes or disposable syringe-needle units (i.e., the needle is integral to the syringe) shall be used for the injection or aspiration of other potentially infectious materials. Extreme caution shall be used when handling needles and syringes. A needle shall not be bent, sheared, replaced in the sheath or guard, or removed from the syringe following use. The needle and syringe shall be promptly placed in a puncture-resistant container and autoclaved or decontaminated before reuse or disposal. (K) All spills shall be immediately contained and cleaned up by appropriate professional staff or others properly trained and equipped to work with potentially concentrated infectious materials. (L) A spill or accident that results in an exposure incident shall be immediately reported to the laboratory director or other responsible person. (M) A biosafety manual shall be prepared or adopted and periodically reviewed and updated at least annually or more often if necessary. Personnel shall be advised of potential hazards, shall be required to read instructions on practices and procedures, and shall be required to follow them. (iii) Containment equipment. (A) Certified biological safety cabinets (Class I, II, or III) or other appropriate combinations of personal protection or physical containment devices, such as special protective clothing, respirators, centrifuge safety cups, sealed centrifuge rotors, and containment caging for animals, shall be used for all activities with other potentially infectious materials that pose a threat of exposure to droplets, splashes, spills, or aerosols. (B) Biological safety cabinets shall be certified when installed, whenever they are moved and at least annually. (3) HIV and HBV research laboratories shall meet the following criteria: (I) Each laboratory shall contain a facility for hand washing and an eye wash facility which is readily available within the work area. (ii) An autoclave for decontamination of regulated waste shall be available. (4) HIV and HBV production facilities shall meet the following criteria: (I) The work areas shall be separated from areas that are open to unrestricted traffic flow within the building. Passage through two sets of doors shall be the basic requirement for entry into the work area from access corridors or other contiguous areas. Physical separation of the high-containment work area from access corridors or other areas or activities may also be provided by a double-doored clothes-change room (showers may be included), airlock, or other access facility that requires passing through two sets of doors before entering the work area. (ii) The surfaces of doors, walls, floors and ceilings in the work area shall be water resistant so that they can be easily cleaned. Penetrations in these surfaces shall be sealed or capable of being sealed to facilitate decontamination. (iii) Each work area shall contain a sink for washing hands and a readily available eye wash facility. The sink shall be foot, elbow, or automatically operated and shall be located near the exit door of the work area. (iv) Access doors to the work area or containment module shall be self-closing. (v) An autoclave for decontamination of regulated waste shall be available within or as near as possible to the work area. (vi) A ducted exhaust-air ventilation system shall be provided. This system shall create directional airflow that draws air into the work area through the entry area. The exhaust air shall not be recirculated to any other area of the building, shall be discharged to the outside, and shall be dispersed away from occupied areas and air intakes. The proper direction of the airflow shall be verified (i.e., into the work area). (5) Training Requirements. Additional training requirements for employees in HIV and HBV research laboratories and HIV and HBV production facilities are specified in paragraph (g)(2)(ix).

(f) Hepatitis B vaccination and post-exposure evaluation and follow-up -
(1) General. (I) The employer shall make available the hepatitis B vaccine and vaccination series to all employees who have occupational exposure, and post-exposure evaluation and follow-up to all employees who have had an exposure incident. (ii) The employer shall ensure that all medical evaluations and procedures including the hepatitis B vaccine and vaccination series and post-exposure evaluation and follow-up, including prophylaxis, are: (A) Made available at no cost to the employee; (B) Made available to the employee at a reasonable time and place; (C) Performed by or under the supervision of a licensed physician or by or under the supervision of another licensed healthcare

professional; and (D) Provided according to recommendations of the U.S. Public Health Service current at the time these evaluations and procedures take place, except as specified by this paragraph (f). (iii) The employer shall ensure that all laboratory tests are conducted by an accredited laboratory at no cost to the employee.

(2) Hepatitis B Vaccination. (I) Hepatitis B vaccination shall be made available after the employee has received the training required in paragraph (g)(2)(vii)(I) and within 10 working days of initial assignment to all employees who have occupational exposure unless the employee has previously received the complete hepatitis B vaccination series, antibody testing has revealed that the employee is immune, or the vaccine is contraindicated for medical reasons. (ii) The employer shall not make participation in a prescreening program a prerequisite for receiving hepatitis B vaccination. (iii) If the employee initially declines hepatitis B vaccination but at a later date while still covered under the standard decides to accept the vaccination, the employer shall make available hepatitis B vaccination at that time. (iv) The employer shall assure that employees who decline to accept hepatitis B vaccination offered by the employer sign the statement in appendix A. (v) If a routine booster dose(s) of hepatitis B vaccine is recommended by the U.S. Public Health Service at a future date, such booster dose(s) shall be made available in accordance with section (f)(1)(ii).

(3) Post-exposure Evaluation and Follow-up. Following a report of an exposure incident, the employer shall make immediately available to the exposed employee a confidential medical evaluation and follow-up, including at least the following elements: (I) Documentation of the route(s) of exposure, and the circumstances under which the exposure incident occurred; (ii) Identification and documentation of the source individual, unless the employer can establish that identification is infeasible o prohibited by state or local law; (A) The source individual's blood shall be tested as soon as feasible and after consent is obtained in order to determine HBV and HIV infectivity. If consent is not obtained, the employer shall establish that legally required consent cannot be obtained. When the source individual's consent is not required by law, the source individual's blood, if available, shall be tested and the results documented. (B) When the source individual is already known to be infected with HBV or HIV, testing for the source individual's known HBV or HIV status need not be repeated. (C) Results of the source individual's testing shall be made available to the exposed employee, and the employee shall be informed of applicable laws and regulations concerning disclosure of the identity and infectious status of the source individual. (iii) Collection and testing of blood for HBV and HIV serological status; (A) The exposed employee's blood shall be collected as soon as feasible and tested after consent is obtained. (B) If the employee consents to baseline blood collection, but does not give consent at that time for HIV serologic testing, the sample shall be preserved for at least 90 days. If, within 90 days of the exposure incident, the employee elects to have the baseline sample tested, such testing shall be done as soon as feasible. (iv) Post-exposure prophylaxis, when medically indicated, as recommended by the U.S. Public Health Service; (v) Counseling; and (vi) Evaluation of reported illnesses.

(4) Information Provided to the Healthcare Professional. (I) The employer shall ensure that the healthcare professional responsible for the employee's Hepatitis B vaccination is provided a copy of this regulation. (ii) The employer shall ensure that the healthcare professional evaluating an employee after an exposure incident is provided the following information: (A) A copy of this regulation; (B) A description of the exposed employee's duties as they relate to the exposure incident; (C) Documentation of the route(s) of exposure and circumstances under which exposure occurred; (D) Results of the source individual's blood testing, if available; and (E) All medical records relevant to the appropriate treatment of the employee including vaccination status which are the employer's responsibility to maintain.

(5) Healthcare Professional's Written Opinion. The employer shall obtain and provide the employee with a copy of the evaluating healthcare professional's written opinion within 15 days of the completion of the evaluation. (I) The healthcare professional's written opinion for Hepatitis B vaccination shall be limited to whether Hepatitis B vaccination is indicated for an employee, and if the employee has received such vaccination. (ii) The healthcare professional's written opinion for post-exposure evaluation and follow-up shall be limited to the following information: (A) That the employee has been informed of the results of the evaluation; and (B) That the employee has been told about any medical conditions resulting from exposure to blood or other potentially infectious materials which require further evaluation or treatment. (iii) All other findings or diagnoses shall remain confidential and shall not be included in the written report. (6) Medical Recordkeeping. Medical records required by this standard shall be maintained in accordance with paragraph (h)(1) of this section.

(g) Communication of hazards to employees - (1) Labels and signs. (I) Labels. (A) Warning labels shall be affixed to containers of regulated waste, refrigerators and freezers containing blood or other potentially infectious material; and other containers used to store, transport or ship blood or other potentially infectious materials, except as provided in paragraph (g)(1)(I)(E), (F) and (G). (B) Labels required by this section shall include the following legend:

*** ILLUSTRATION OMITTED ***

(C) These labels shall be fluorescent orange or orange-red or predominantly so, with lettering and symbols in a contrasting color. (D) Labels shall be affixed as close as feasible to the container by string, wire, adhesive, or other method that prevents their loss or unintentional removal. (E) Red bags or red containers may be substituted for labels. (F) Containers of blood, blood components, or blood products that are labeled as to their contents and have been released for transfusion or other clinical use are exempted from the labeling requirements of paragraph (g). (G) Individual containers of blood or other potentially infectious materials that are placed in a labeled container during storage, transport, shipment or disposal are exempted from the labeling requirement. (H) Labels required for contaminated equipment shall be in accordance with this paragraph and shall also state which portions of the equipment remain contaminated. (I) Regulated waste that has been decontaminated need not be labeled or color-coded. (ii) Signs. (A)

The employer shall post signs at the entrance to work areas specified in paragraph (e), HIV and HBV Research Laboratory and Production Facilities, which shall bear the following legend:

*** ILLUSTRATION OMITTED ***

(Name of the Infectious Agent)
(Special requirements for entering the area)
(Name, telephone number of the laboratory director or other responsible person.)
(B) These signs shall be fluorescent orange-red or predominantly so, with lettering and symbols in a contrasting color.

(2) Information and Training. (I) Employers shall ensure that all employees with occupational exposure participate in a training program which must be provided at no cost to the employee and during working hours. (ii) Training shall be provided as follows: (A) At the time of initial assignment to tasks where occupational exposure may take place; (B) Within 90 days after the effective date of the standard; and (C) At least annually thereafter. (iii) For employees who have received training on bloodborne pathogens in the year preceding the effective date of the standard, only training with respect to the provisions of the standard which were not included need be provided. (iv) Annual training for all employees shall be provided within one year of their previous training. (v) Employers shall provide additional training when changes such as modification of tasks or procedures or institution of new tasks or procedures affect the employee's occupational exposure. The additional training may be limited to addressing the new exposures created. (vi) Material appropriate in content and vocabulary to educational level, literacy, and language of employees shall be used. (vii) The training program shall contain at a minimum the following elements: (A) An accessible copy of the regulatory text of this standard and an explanation of its contents; (B) A general explanation of the epidemiology and symptoms of bloodborne diseases; (C) An explanation of the modes of transmission of bloodborne pathogens; (D) An explanation of the employer's exposure control plan and the means by which the employee can obtain a copy of the written plan; (E) An explanation of the appropriate methods for recognizing tasks and other activities that may involve exposure to blood and other potentially infectious materials; (F) An explanation of the use and limitations of methods that will prevent or reduce exposure including appropriate engineering controls, work practices, and personal protective equipment; (G) Information on the types, proper use, location, removal, handling, decontamination and disposal of personal protective equipment; (H) An explanation of the basis for selection of personal protective equipment; (I) Information on the hepatitis B vaccine, including information on its efficacy, safety, method of administration, the benefits of being vaccinated, and that the vaccine and vaccination will be offered free of charge; (J) Information on the appropriate actions to take and persons to contact in an emergency involving blood or other potentially infectious materials; (K) An explanation of the procedure to follow if an exposure incident occurs, including the method of reporting the incident and the medical follow-up that will be made available; (L) Information on the post-exposure evaluation and follow-up that the employer is required to provide for the

employee following an exposure incident; (M) An explanation of the signs and labels and/or color coding required by paragraph (g)(1); and (N) An opportunity for interactive questions and answers with the person conducting the training session. (viii) The person conducting the training shall be knowledgeable in the subject matter covered by the elements contained in the training program as it relates to the workplace that the training will address. (ix) Additional Initial Training for Employees in HIV and HBV Laboratories and Production Facilities. Employees in HIV or HBV research laboratories and HIV or HBV production facilities shall receive the following initial training in addition to the above training requirements. (A) The employer shall assure that employees demonstrate proficiency in standard microbiological practices and techniques and in the practices and operations specific to the facility before being allowed to work with HIV or HBV. (B) The employer shall assure that employees have prior experience in the handling of human pathogens or tissue cultures before working with HIV or HBV. (C) The employer shall provide a training program to employees who have no prior experience in handling human pathogens. Initial work activities shall not include the handling of infectious agents. A progression of work activities shall be assigned as techniques are learned and proficiency is developed. The employer shall assure that employees participate in work activities involving infectious agents only after proficiency has been demonstrated.

(h) Recordkeeping - (1) Medical Records. (I) The employer shall establish and maintain an accurate record for each employee with occupational exposure, in accordance with 29 CFR 1910.20. (ii) This record shall include: (A) The name and social security number of the employee; (B) A copy of the employee's hepatitis B vaccination status including the dates of all the hepatitis B vaccinations and any medical records relative to the employee's ability to receive vaccination as required by paragraph (f)(2); (C) A copy of all results of examinations, medical testing, and follow-up procedures as required by paragraph (f)(3); (D) The employer's copy of the healthcare professional's written opinion as required by paragraph (f)(5); and (E) A copy of the information provided to the healthcare professional as required by paragraphs (f)(4)(ii)(B)(C) and (D). (iii) Confidentiality. The employer shall ensure that employee medical records required by paragraph (h)(1) are: (A) Kept confidential; and (B) Not disclosed or reported without the employee's express written consent to any person within or outside the workplace except as required by this section or as may be required by law. (iv) The employer shall maintain the records required by paragraph (h) for at least the duration of employment plus 30 years in accordance with 29 CFR 1910.20. (2) Training Records. (I) Training records shall include the following information: (A) The dates of the training sessions;
(B) The contents or a summary of the training sessions; (C) The names and qualifications of persons conducting the training; and (D) The names and job titles of all persons attending the training sessions. (ii) Training records shall be maintained for 3 years from the date on which the training occurred. (3) Availability. (I) The employer shall ensure that all records required to be maintained by this section shall be made available upon request to the Assistant Secretary and the Director for examination and copying. (ii) Employee training records required by this paragraph shall be provided upon request for

examination and copying to employees, to employee representatives, to the Director, and to the Assistant Secretary. (iii) Employee medical records required by this paragraph shall be provided upon request for examination and copying to the subject employee, to anyone having written consent of the subject employee, to the Director, and to the Assistant Secretary in accordance with 29 CFR 1910.20. (4) Transfer of Records. (I) The employer shall comply with the requirements involving transfer of records set forth in 29 CFR 1910.20(h). (ii) If the employer ceases to do business and there is no successor employer to receive and retain the records for the prescribed period, the employer shall notify the Director, at least three months prior to their disposal and transmit them to the Director, if required by the Director to do so, within that three month period.

(i) Dates - (1) Effective Date. The standard shall become effective on March 6, 1992. (2) The Exposure Control Plan required by paragraph (C) of this section shall be completed on or before May 5, 1992. (3) Paragraph (g)(2) Information and Training and (h) Recordkeeping shall take effect on or before June 4, 1992. (4) Paragraphs (d)(2) Engineering and Work Practice Controls, (d)(3) Personal Protective Equipment, (d)(4) Housekeeping, (e) HIV and HBV Research Laboratories and Production Facilities, (f) Hepatitis B Vaccination and Post-Exposure Evaluation and Follow-up, and (g) (1) Labels and Signs, shall take effect July 6, 1992.

RESOURCES

Resources are offered for the information of readers. The author and publisher neither endorse nor warranty any product or vendor.

Government Agency Web Sites

ADA	gopher://justice12.usdoj.gov:70/11/crt/ada
Centers Disease Control	http://www.cdc.gov
Fish & Wildlife Service	http://www.fws.gov
FDA	http://www.fda.gov
FDA CDRH	http://www.fda.gov/cdrh
Internet Medline	http://igm.nlm.nih.gov
NIOSH	http://www.cdc.gov/niosh/homepage.html
OSHA	http://www.osha.gov

MSDS Resources
Links to MSDS listings:
http://www.safetyplace.com/library/linkmsds.html

Charting & Transcription Software
Notes Express ™   (800) 542-4476
http://www.notesexpress.com

Telephone Triage Software
Healthline Systems Inc.　　(800) 733-8737
http://www.healthlinesystems.com　　Sharp Focus® for Windows®

Primus Systems Inc.　　(508) 481-9171
http://www.primusmed.com　　Telephone Triage™ software

Interviewing & Hiring Software
Coremedia Training Solutions Inc.　　(800) 537-8352
1732 NW Quimby St. Ste.201　　SmartHire® for Windows®
Portland OR 97209

Acupuncture Business Forms
Mission Printing　　(209) 227-7640
3 E. Shields Avenue
Fresno, CA 93704

Acupuncture Professional Liability Insurance
Lincoln Associates Ltd.　　(800) 860-8330
188 Industrial Dr. Suite 226　　(630) 833-0900
Elmhurst, IL 60126

Acupuncture Risk Management Seminars & Videos
David Kailin, L Ac, MPH　　(541) 757-8601
CMS Press　　bloodborne pathogen & hazard
P.O.Box 2115　　communication training & videos;
Corvallis, OR 97339　　forms, publications, seminars.

Acupuncture Supplies
Helio Medical Supplies Inc.　　(800) 672-2726
2080-A Walsh Avenue　　source for disposable needles,
Santa Clara, CA 95050　　infra-red lamps, etc.

Lhasa Medical Inc. (800) 722-8775
539 Accord Stn. source for disposable needles,
Accord, MA 02018 etc.

OMS Medical Supplies Inc. (800) 323-1839
1959 Washington St. source for disposable needles,
Braintree, MA 02184 microcurrent TENS units, etc.

Microcurrent TENS Devices
OMS Medical Supplies Inc. (800) 323-1839
1959 Washington St. Micro 300; Micro 850
Braintree, MA 02184

MicroStim, Inc. (800) 326-9119
8333 W.McNab Rd., #222 MicroStim 100, MicroStim 400
Tamarac, FL 33321

Microcurrent Research, Inc. (800) 872-6789
3810 E. Desert Cove Ave. Acutron Mentor
Phoenix, AZ 85028

Lasers
Boston Chinese Medicine (617) 720-4448
http://www.acupuncture.com/Acup/Naeser2.htm
source for Naeser & Wei text: LASER ACUPUNCTURE

Control Optics Corp. (818) 813-1991
1311 Brooks Dr. Ste.J source for laser eyeshields
Baldwin Park, CA 91706

Kentek Corp. (800) 432-2323
19 Depot St. source for laser eyeshields
Pittsfield, NH 03263

Laser Institute of America   (800) 34-LASER
http://www.creol.ucf.edu/~lia/home.html
12424 Research Parkway   source for ANSI Z136.1 laser
Suite # 125   standards, laser training texts
Orlando, FL 32826   & videos

Rockwell Laser Industries, Inc.   LaserNet®
http://www.rli.com   laser safety info & database

Univ. of Illinois at Urbana-Champaign,   Radiation Safety Section
http://.phantom.ehs.uiuc.edu/~rad/laser/   laser safety info

Magnets
Total Health   (800) 283-2833
http://hre.com/totalhealth/magindex.html
170 Fulton St.
Farmingdale, NY 11735   magnetic field therapy home page

Albert Roy Davis Research Laboratory
Scientific Research & Development
P.O.Box 655   info on experimental use of
Green Cover Springs, FL 32043   magnets in healing

BIBLIOGRAPHY

Chapter 1 Dimensions of Risk & Benefit

p.13   Porter-O'Grady, T. 1996 Oct. 18, Salishan Lodge, Gleneden, OR   Seminar notes

Chapter 2 Scope of Risk Management

p.21   Head 1989 ESSENTIALS OF RISK CONTROL, Vol.I, 2nd Ed. Insurance Institute of America, Malvern PA

p.23   Anon 1996 telephone interview, proprietary business data

p.24   Norheim & Fonnebo 1995 Adverse effects of acupuncture. Lancet 345(8958):1175

Chapter 4 Physical Plant

p.32   DOJ 1992 The Americans With Disabilities Act - Questions and Answers   rev. Sept. gopher://justice2.usdoj.gov:70/00/crt/ada/ada.dos

p.32   CBBBF 1995 Professional Offices - Access Equals Opportunity - Your Guide To The ADA. Council of Better Business Bureau's Fndtn. Arlington VA p.33 NRH 1994 The ADA - Answers to Questions Commonly Asked by Hospitals and Health Care Providers. National Rehabilitation Hospital Wash.D.C.

p.35 Uppsala Univ. Hosp. 1997 Dept. Occup. & Envir. Hlth. http://www2.uu.se/insts/arbmilj/indoor.html

p.35 OSHA 1995 Technical Manual II:2 Indoor Air Quality Investigation http:www.osha-slc.gov/TechMan_data/TM16.html

p.35 OSHA 1995 op.cit.

p.39 OR.OSHA 1995 Fire Protection Using Portable Fire Extinguishers - Fact Sheet 8/15/95 Consultative Services Section, Oregon Occupational Safety & Health Div.

Chapter 5   Employers & Employees

p.49 Arthur 1995 MANAGING HUMAN RESOURCES IN SMALL & MID-SIZED COMPANIES 2nd Ed. AMACOM San Francisco

p.49 USDOJ 1992 Sept. ADA- QUESTIONS & ANSWERS gopher://justice2.usdoj.gov:70/00/crt/ada/ada.dos

p.51 Arthur 1995 ibid

p.51 Dickson 1995 LAW IN THE HEALTH AND HUMAN SERVICES Free Press NY p.52   Harper Business 1990 THE COMPANY POLICY MANUAL Management Resources Inc. NY

p.53   OSHA 1997 June 27 http://www.osha-slc.gov/ergo/

Chapter 6   Bloodborne Pathogens

p.57   OSHA 1996
http://www.osha.gov/oshFAQs/pathogens1.html

p.57   MMWR 1989 Guidelines for Prevention of Transmission of Human Immunodeficiency Virus and Hepatitis B Virus to Health Care and Public Safety Workers. 38(S-6)
http://aepo-xdv-www.epo.cdc.gov/wonder/prevguid/tp_01493.htm

p.60   OSHA 1994 Occupational Exposure To Bloodborne Pathogens - Interpretive Quips (IQ's), Jan. 1994 Version

p.61   CDC 1997 Sterilization or Disinfection of Patient-Care Equipment: General Principles
http://www.cdc.gov/ncidod/diseases/hip/sterilgp.htm

p.61   NAF 1997 CLEAN NEEDLE TECHNIQUE MANUAL FOR ACUPUNCTURISTS 4th Ed. Wash. D.C. National Acupuncture Foundation   p.30-1

p.62   CDC 1985 Guideline For Handwashing And Hospital Environmental Control p.7; in: USDHHS 1988

p.62   CDC 1985 ibid

p.63   USDHHS 1988 GUIDELINES FOR PROTECTING THE SAFETY AND HEALTH OF HEALTH CARE WORKERS U.S. Department Health & Human Services DHHS (NIOSH) Publication 88-119

p.63   NAF 1997 op.cit.

p.65   CDC 1997a
http://www.cdc.gov/od/ohs/manual/pprotect.htm

p.65   CDC 1997b
http://www.cdc.gov/travel/yellowbk/page154.htm

p.65   NIOSH 1997 http://www.cdc.gov/niosh/latexalt.html

p.69   MMWR 1989 ibid

p.69   CD Summary 1996 New Guidelines For Prophylaxis Following Occupational Exposure to HIV v.45, #12, 6/11/96 Center for Disease Prevention & Epidemiology, Oregon Health Div., Dept. Human Resources, Portland OR

Chapter 7   Records & Billing

p.77   AHIMA 1992 PRINCIPLES OF MEDICAL RECORD DOCUMENTATION Chicago

p.77   JCAHO 1995 ACCREDITATION MANUAL FOR HOSPITALS Chicago

p.79   Seidel et al 1991 MOSBY'S GUIDE TO PHYSICAL EXAMINATION 2nd Ed. St.Louis Ch.20

p.91   OMA 1994 THE MEDICO-LEGAL HANDBOOK Oregon Medical Assn. p.73

p.92   AMA 1996a PHYSICIANS' CURRENT PROCEDURAL TERMINOLOGY (CPT 1996) 4th Ed. Revised Chicago

p.92   CSOM 1997a telephone interview, Neal Miller, California Society Oriental Medicine

p.94   CSOM 1997b http://www.quickcom.net/csom

p.95   AMA 1996b INTERNATIONAL CLASSIFICATION OF DISEASES, 9th Rev. Clin. Modifictn., 4th Ed. (ICD 9 CM)

Chapter 8   Medical Advice

p.99   OMA 1994 op.cit. p.9

p.99   McWay 1997 LEGAL ASPECTS OF HEALTH INFORMATION MANAGEMENT Delmar Pub. San Francisco

p.100   Alton 1977 op.cit. p.25

p.107   OMA 1994 op.cit. p.43

p.109   Kleinman 1980 PATIENTS AND HEALERS IN THE CONTEXT OF CULTURE U. Cal. Press Berkeley Ch.3

Chapter 9 Medical Emergencies

p.111 Bergeron, J.D. 1982 1ST RESPONDER 2nd Ed. Prentice Hall, Englewood Cliffs NJ

p.111 Malamed, S.F. 1987 HANDBOOK OF MEDICAL EMERGENCIES IN THE DENTAL OFFICE 3rd Ed. C.V. Mosby Co. St.Louis

Chapter 10 Interpersonal Aspects of Treatment

p.118 Novack 1987 Therapeutic aspects of the clinical encounter. J.Genl.Int.Med. Sept/Oct 2:346-55

p.118 Meissner 1992 The concept of the therapeutic alliance. J.Amer.Psychoanal.Assoc. 40(4)1059-87

p.119 Rosenzweig 1993 Emergency Rapport. J.Emerg.Med. 11:775-8

p.122 OR BME 1997 Sexual Boundary Allegations: BME 1991-1996 in: BME Report, Sp/Sum Issue

Chapter 11 Legal Aspects of Treatment

p.127 OR BME 1997 Memorandum 8/14 RE: Use of Titles by Oregon Licensed Acupuncturists

p.128 McWay 1997 op.cit. p.40

p.130 Sloan 1992 PROFESSIONAL MALPRACTICE Oceana Pub., Dobbs Ferry NY

p.132 McWay 1997 op.cit. p.41

p.134 OMA 1994 op.cit. p.94

Chapter 12   FDA Regulations

p.144 FDA 1996a Compliance Policy Guide, Sec. 120.500 Aug.1996

p.145 FDA 1996b Compliance Policy Guide, Sec.305.100 Aug.1996

p.146 CAAOM 1997 SCOPE OF PRACTICE FOR LICENSED ACUPUNCTURISTS ver.2.5 March   Santa Barbara, CA (805) 957-4384

p.147 Fed.Register 1996 12/6 v.61 #236 pp.64616-64617

Chapter 13   Technical Aspects of Treatment

p.153 CDC 1993 May 28 Recommended Infection Control Practices For Dentistry (PDF-181K) Vol. 42, No. RR-8

p.157 MMWR 1993 Recommendedd Infection Control Practices For Dentistry   42(RR-8)
http://www.cdc.gov/nccdphp/oh/icbbp.htm

Chapter 14 Acupuncture Needles

p.160 Davis & Powell 1985 Auricular perichondritis secondary to acupuncture. Arch.Otolaryngology 111(11):770-1

p.160 Lee & McIlwain 1985 Subacute bacterial endocarditis following ear acupuncture. Intl.J.Cardiology 7(1):62-3

p.160 Gilbert 1987 Auricular complications of acupuncture. N.Z.Med.J. 100(819): 141-2

p.160 Sorensen 1990 Auricular perichondritis caused by acupuncture therapy. Ugeskrift for Laeger 152(11):752-3

p.161 Stryker et al 1986 Outbreak of hepatitis B associated with acupuncture. J.Fam.Pract. 22(2):155-8

p.161 Kent et al 1988 A large outbreak of acupuncture-associated hepatitis B. Amer.J.Epi. 127(3):591-8

p.161 Slater et al 1988 An acupuncture-associated outbreak of hepatitis B on Jerusalem. Euro.J.Epi. 4(3):322-5

p.161 CDR Weekly 1992 Hepatitis B associated with an acupuncture clinic. Communicable Dis. Report 2(48):219

p.164 NAF 1997 op.cit.

p.166 Huet et al 1990 Unrecognized pneumothorax after acupuncture in a female patient with anorexia nervosa. Presse Medicale 19(30):1415 p.166 Gray et al 1991 Pneumothorax resulting from acupuncture. Can.Assn.Radiol.J. 42(2):139-40

p.166 Devouassoux et al 1994 Bilateral pneumothorax of unusual origin. Rev. de Pneumologie Clinique 50(4):186-7

p.166 Norheim 1994 Adverse effects of acupuncture - a study of the literature from 1981-92. Tidsskrift for Den Norske Laegeforening 114(10):1192-94

p.166 Norheim & Fonnebo 1995 Adverse effects of acupuncture. Lancet 345(8958):1175

p.167 Holland 1989 CROSS SECTIONAL ATLAS OF COMMONLY USED ACUPUNCTURE POINTS OF THE ARM AND LEG Holland, NIAOM Seattle

p.167 Galutin & Autin 1988 Permanent subcutaneous acupuncture needles: radiographic manifestations. Can.Assn.Rad.J. 39(1):54-6

p.167 Hasegawa et al 1990 Acupuncture needles straying in the central nervous system and presenting neurological signs and symptoms. Rinsho Shinkeigaku 30(10):1109-13

p.167 Murata et al 1990 Subarachnoid hemorrhage and spinal root injury caused by acupuncture needle - case report. Neurologia Medico-Chirurgica 30(12):956-9

p.167 Sakai et al 1994 Removal of a retained acupuncture needle in the paraspinal muscle using a neuronavigator. Plast.& Reconstruct.Surg. 94(7):1097-8 p.167   Southworth & Hartwig 1990 Foreign body in the median nerve: a complication of acupuncture. J.Hand Surg- British 15(1):111-2

p.167   Gi et al 1994 Spinal cord stab injury by acupuncture needle: a case report. No Shinkei Geka 22(2):151-4

Chapter 15   Moxibustion

p.182   So 1977 A COMPLETE COURSE IN CHINESE ACUPUNCTURE New Engl. Schl. Acup. Watertown MA

Chapter 18   Herbs & Dietary Supplements

p.209   FDA 1991 Import Alert #66-10
http://www.fda.gov/ora/fiars/ora_import_ia6610.html

p.209   CSOM 1997 http://www.quickcom.net/csom/

p.209   CA Dept.Hlth.Svcs. 1992 Common Toxic Ingredients Found In Asian Patent Medicines. State of CA 1/28 p.1

p.210   FDA 1991 ibid

p.210   Espinoza et al 1995 Arsenic and mercury in traditional Chinese herbal balls. NEJM 333:803-4

p.211   F&WS 1996 Endangered & threatened species used in oriental medicine. Fish & Wildlife Service, conference handout. See: http://www.fws.gov/r9dia/temproc.html

p.212 Gordon 1995 Chapparal ingestion. JAMA 273(6):489-90

p.212 Winship 1991 Toxicity of comfrey. Adverse Drug React Toxicl Rev 10(1):47-59

p.212 Couet et al 1996 Analysis, separation, and bioassay of pyrrolizidine alkaloids from comfrey (Symphytum officinale). Nat Toxins 4(4):163-7

p.212 MMWR 1996 Morbidity & MortalityWeekly Report 8/16 45(32):689-92

p.212 FDA 1997a http://vm.cfsan.fda.gov/~lrd/fr97064a.html

p.212 Marandino 1997 Ephedra falls under FDA jurisdiction. Vegetarian Times, Sept. p.18-20

p.212 Tao & Bolger 1997 Hazard assessment of germanium supplements. Regul.Toxicol.Pharmacol. 25(3):211-19

p.212 FDA 1996 What information is known about the availability of L-tryptophan. Ctr.Food Safety & Applied Nutrition http://vm.cfsan.fda.gov/~dms/ds-tryp1.html

p.212 Olson 1996 Benefits and liabilities of vitamin A and carotenoids. J.Nutr. 126(4Suppl):1208S-12S

p.212 Polifka et al 1996 Clinical teratology counseling and consultation report: high dose beta-carotene use during early pregnancy. Teratology 54(2): 103-7 p.213   FDA 1997b FDA warns consumers against dietary supplement products that may contain digitalis mislabeled as 'plantain'. FDA Press Office 6/12 http://www.fda.gov/bbs/topics/NEWS/NEW00570.html

p.215   Anon 1996 personal communication

p.215   Bensky et al 1986 CHINESE HERBAL MEDICINE MATERIA MEDICA Eastland Press Seattle

p.215   Chen 1997 Recognition And Prevention Of Herb-Drug Interactions Cal.J.Or.Med. Sept. p.9-11

p.215   DFC 1998 DRUG FACTS AND COMPARISONS 1998 Ed. Lippincott-Raven Pub. St.Louis

Chapter 20   Electroacupuncture

p.228   Naeser & Wei 1994 op.cit. p.39

p.228   NAF 1997 op.cit. p.43

p.228   OMS 1996 OMS Medical Supplies Catalog, Braintree, MA p.41

p.229   NAF 1997 ibid.

p.229   CCAOM 1997 op.cit. p.24

Chapter 21 Laser Devices

p.236 OSHA 1995 Technical Manual, Section II, Ch.6

p.236 Naeser & Wei 1994 op.cit. part 1, p.2

p.236 Naeser & Wei 1994 op.cit. p.3

p.238 ANSI 1993 American National Standard for the Safe Use of Lasers ANSI Z136.1 Laser Institute of America Orlando, FL

p.238 ANSI 1996 American National Standard for the Safe Use of Lasers in Health Care Facilities ANSI Z136.3 Laser Institute of America Orlando, FL

p.238 Rockwell 1996 Rockwell Laser Industries, Inc. Laser Accident Database http://www.rli.com/accident

p.241 CAAOM 1997 op.cit. p.44

Chapter 22 Magnetic Devices

p.245 Total Health 1997 http://hre.com/totalhealth/magindex.html

p.245 Becker 1990 CROSS CURRENTS Tarcher NY p.144

INDEX

abandonment	128
accountability	12
acupressure, best practices	225
bloodborne pathogen	219
excess pressure	221
improper touch	222
ADA, access	32
hiring	49
advice, initial	99
scope	103
ANSI	238
autoclave	154
best practices	152, 173, 185, 194, 205, 217, 225, 233, 243, 249
billing, collection	91
ethics	89
limits	86
biohazard labeling	72
bloodborne pathogen	57, 152, 156, 160, 189, 199, 219, 297
engineering controls	61
exposure control plan	58, 273
exposure incident	69, 270-2
exposure risk determination	59
HBV vaccination	68, 267
recordkeeping	74
training	72
work practices	61, 64
building security	31

chemical hazard, communication	41, 265, 281
labeling	47
training	44
codes, diagnostic	94
procedure	92
coining, best practices	205
bloodborne pathogen	199
technical notes	197
mis-attribution	202
conditions of work	55
critical instruments	153
cupping, best practices	194
bloodborne pathogen	189
technical notes	187
decontamination, table	156
dietary supplements	(see herbs)
disinfection, equipment	152
DSHEA	149, 207
duty, employers	47
professional	127
electrical system	33
electroacupuncture, best practices	233
FDA compliance	229
technical notes	227
emergencies, medical	111
emergency action plan	37, 253
ergonomics	53
ethics	9
fainting	113
fall injury	36
FDA, medical device class	141

FDA standards	141
acupuncture devices	147
dietary supplements	149
fire prevention plan	39, 256
firing, employee	50
first aid, limits	114
fraud, medical	128, 144
fumes	35
glutaraldehyde	153
guarantees of outcome	104
handwashing	62
harms, material	23
hazard communication, chemical	41, 265, 281
hepatitis B virus (HBV)	57, 68, 267
hepatitis C virus (HCV)	57
herbs, adulteration	208
adverse events	215
best practices	217
compounding	213
injurious	211
labeling	207, 214
quality	214
hiring	48
HIV	57
housekeeping	66
HVAC	33
hygienic practices	156
identification, professional	127
informed consent	105
investigational device	143

labeled use	143
labeling, biohazard	72
chemical hazard	43
diagnostic & prognostic	108
herbs	207, 214
laser hazard	235
laser, best practices	243
hazard classes	235
hazard control	238
regulations & standards	241
technical notes	235
latex, allergy	65
permeability	65
laundry, contaminated	67
magnets, best practices	249
FDA regulation	246
technical notes	245
malpractice	132
medical record, confidentiality	81
contents	77
destruction	85
employee	74, 268
release	81, 269
retention	85
modesty	120
moral community	10
moxibustion, best practices	185
direct	181-3
indirect	177, 179
MSDS	42, 258
needles, accountability	159
best practices	173

needles, bloodborne pathogen	160
manufacturing flaws	168
structural damage	165
travel kit	170
negligence	130
non-standard medicine	138
off-label use	143
OPIM	57
OSHA, 200 form	48
bloodborne pathogen	(see bloodborne pathogen)
chemical hazard communication	41, 265, 281
emergency action plan	37, 253
job safety & health poster	47
particulates	35
personal protective equipment	(see PPE)
policies, employers	52
PPE	64, 113, 156, 162, 189-91, 199, 219, 222, 240
primary care	134
privacy	120
procedures, employers	52
rapport	119
relationship, fiduciary	122
patient/practitioner	99
professional	109
therapeutic	117
reporting requirements	82, 128
risk, cascade	14
contexts	27
dimensions	13
management	19

risk, selection 21

scope of practice 94, 103, 125
sexual boundaries 121, 222
standards of care 138
sterilization, equipment 152

technical guidelines 151
telephone protocol 100
TENS 147, 228, 230
termination, employee 50
torts 128
training, bloodborne pathogen 72
       chemical hazard communication 44
       emergency evacuation 38
       fire prevention 39
transference 118
travel kit 170
treatment limits 86

universal precautions 60
un-labeled device 143

vaccination, HBV 68, 267

waste, regulated 67
    contaminated 68

Notes

CMS Press

The Source For Acupuncture-Specific Safety Training Videos:
> Acupuncture Bloodborne Pathogens
> Chemical Hazard Communication

On-Line Catalog:
> http://www.convergentmedical.com

Orders:
> (541) 757-8601
> P.O. Box 2115
> Corvallis, OR 97339 USA